INTERVENTIONAL CARDIOLOGY CLINICS

www.interventional.theclinics.com

Editor-in-Chief

MATTHEW J. PRICE

Transcatheter Mitral Valve Intervention

January 2016 • Volume 5 • Number 1

Editor

JASON H. ROGERS

ELSEVIER

1600 John F. Kennedy Boulevard • Suite 1800 • Philadelphia, Pennsylvania, 19103-2899

http://www.theclinics.com

INTERVENTIONAL CARDIOLOGY CLINICS Volume 5, Number 1
January 2016 ISSN 2211-7458, ISBN-13: 978-0-323-41454-8

Editor: Lauren Boyle
Developmental Editor: Susan Showalter

Interventional Cardiology Clinics (ISSN 2211-7458) is published quarterly by Elsevier Inc., 360 Park Avenue South, New York, NY 10010-1710. Months of issue are January, April, July, and October. Subscription prices are USD 195 per year for US individuals, USD 436 for US institutions, USD 100 per year for US students, USD 195 per year for Canadian individuals, USD 520 for Canadian institutions, USD 150 per year for Canadian students, USD 295 per year for international individuals, USD 520 for international institutions, and USD 150 per year for international students. To receive student/resident rate, orders must be accompanied by name of affiliated institution, date of term, and the *signature* of program/residency coordinator on institution letterhead. Orders will be billed at individual rate until proof of status is received. Foreign air speed delivery is included in all *Clinics* subscription prices. All prices are subject to change without notice. **POSTMASTER:** Send address changes to *Interventional Cardiology Clinics*, Elsevier Health Sciences Division, Subscription Customer Service, 3251 Riverport Lane, Maryland Heights, MO 63043. **Customer Service: Telephone: 1-800-654-2452** (U.S. and Canada); **1-314-447-8871** (outside U.S. and Canada). **Fax: 1-314-447-8029. E-mail: journalscustomerservice-usa@elsevier.com (for print support); journalsonlinesupport-usa@elsevier.com (for online support).**

Reprints. For copies of 100 or more of articles in this publication, please contact the Commercial Reprints Department, Elsevier Inc., 360 Park Avenue South, New York, NY 10010-1710. Tel.: 212-633-3874; Fax: 212-633-3820; E-mail: reprints@elsevier.com.

CONTRIBUTORS

EDITOR-IN-CHIEF

MATTHEW J. PRICE, MD
Assistant Professor, Scripps Translational
Science Institute; Director of the Cardiac
Catheterization Laboratory, Scripps Green
Hospital, La Jolla, California

EDITOR

JASON H. ROGERS, MD, FACC, FSCAI
Professor of Cardiovascular Medicine;
Director, Interventional Cardiology, University
of California Davis Medical Center,
Sacramento, California

AUTHORS

ALA AL-LAWATI, MD
Division of Cardiothoracic Surgery, St. Paul's
Hospital, University of British Columbia,
Vancouver, British Columbia, Canada

G. ATHAPPAN, MD
Department of Cardiovascular Medicine,
Heart and Vascular Institute, Temple
University Hospital, Philadelphia, Pennsylvania

VASILIS BABALIAROS, MD
Division of Cardiology, Structural Heart and
Valve Center, Emory University School of
Medicine, Atlanta, Georgia

ANSON CHEUNG, MD
Division of Cardiothoracic Surgery, St. Paul's
Hospital, University of British Columbia,
Vancouver, British Columbia, Canada

JOSE F. CONDADO, MD, MS
Division of Cardiology, Structural Heart and
Valve Center, Emory University School of
Medicine, Atlanta, Georgia

TED FELDMAN, MD, FESC, FACC, MSCAI
NorthShore University HealthSystem,
Evanston, Illinois

STEVEN L. GOLDBERG, MD
Rocky Mountain Heart and Lung, Kalispell
Regional Medical Center, Kalispell, Montana;
Chief Medical Officer, Cardiac Dimensions,
Inc, Kirkland, Washington

MAYRA GUERRERO, MD, FACC, FSCAI
NorthShore University HealthSystem,
Evanston, Illinois

CHRISTOPH HAMMERSTINGL, MD
Heart Center University of Bonn, Bonn,
Germany

VLADIMIR JELNIN, MD
Assistant Professor of Cardiology, Division of
Structural and Congenital Heart Disease,
Heart and Vascular Hospital, Hackensack
University Medical Center, Hackensack,
New Jersey

BRIAN KAEBNICK, MD
Division of Cardiology, Structural Heart and
Valve Center, Emory University School of
Medicine, Atlanta, Georgia

SAMIR R. KAPADIA, MD
Professor of Medicine, Director, Cardiac
Catheterization Laboratory, Department of
Cardiovascular Medicine, Heart and Vascular
Institute, Cleveland Clinic, Cleveland, Ohio

CHAD KLIGER, MD
Assistant Professor of Cardiology, Division of
Structural and Congenital Heart Disease,
Department of Cardiothoracic Surgery,
Hofstra University School of Medicine, Lenox
Hill Hospital, North Shore LIJ Health System,
New York, New York

AZEEM LATIB, MD
Interventional Cardiology Unit, EMO-GVM
Centro Cuore Columbus, San Raffaele
Scientific Institute, Milan, Italy

DMITRY B. LEVIN, BA
Research Scientist, Engineer, Division of
Cardiology, Department of Medicine,
University of Washington, Seattle, Washington

JUSTIN P. LEVISAY, MD, FACC, FSCAI
NorthShore University HealthSystem,
Evanston, Illinois

ARJUN MEHTA, MD
NorthShore University HealthSystem,
Evanston, Illinois

JEFFREY M. PAULSEN, MD
Division of Cardiovascular Medicine,
Department of Internal Medicine, University of
California Davis Health System, Sacramento,
California

ELIZABETH M. PERPETUA, DNP, APRN-BC
Faculty Associate, School of Medicine;
Director of Structural Heart Services, Division
of Cardiothoracic Surgery, Department of
Surgery, University of Washington, Seattle,
Washington

MOHAMMAD QASIM RAZA, MD
Department of Cardiovascular Medicine,
Heart and Vascular Institute, Cleveland Clinic,
Cleveland, Ohio

MARK REISMAN, MD
Clinical Professor of Medicine, School of
Medicine; Section Head Interventional
Cardiology, Division of Cardiology,
Department of Medicine, University of
Washington, Seattle, Washington

JASON H. ROGERS, MD, FACC, FSCAI
Professor of Cardiovascular Medicine;
Director, Interventional Cardiology, University
of California Davis Medical Center,
Sacramento, California

CARLOS E. RUIZ, MD, PhD
Professor of Medicine and Pediatrics; Director
of Structural and Congenital Heart Disease
Program, Heart and Vascular Hospital,
Hackensack University Medical Center,
Hackensack, New Jersey

MICHAEL H. SALINGER, MD, FACC, FSCAI
NorthShore University HealthSystem,
Evanston, Illinois

GAGAN D. SINGH, MD
Fellow, Division of Cardiovascular Medicine,
University of California Davis Medical Center,
Sacramento, California

THOMAS W. SMITH, MD, FACC
Assistant Professor of Medicine, Division
of Cardiovascular Medicine, Department of
Internal Medicine, University of California
Davis Health System, Sacramento,
California

PAUL SORAJJA, MD
Director, Center for Valve and Structural Heart
Disease, Minneapolis Heart Institute, Abbott
Northwestern Hospital, Minneapolis,
Minnesota

MAURIZIO TARAMASSO, MD
Department of Cariac Surgery, Herz-Gefäss
Chirurgie, UniversitätsSpital Zürich, Zürich,
Switzerland

FABIO ZUCCHETTA, MD
Cardiac Surgeon, Department of Cardiology,
Thoracic and Vascular Sciences, University of
Padua, Padua, Italy

CONTENTS

 Videos of aortic and subaortic/LVOT flow dynamics accompany this article

Transcatheter mitral valve therapy requires an in-depth understanding of the mitral valve apparatus (annulus, leaflets, chordae tendinae, and papillary muscles) and the impact of various disease states. Adjacent structures (left atrium, left ventricular outflow tract, aortic valve, coronary sinus, and circumflex artery) must also be respected. This article reviews the anatomy and function of the normal and diseased mitral valve apparatus and the implications for catheter-based intervention.

Echocardiography continues to be the most effective imaging tool for the diagnosis and follow-up of mitral valve disease. This review addresses the use of transthoracic echocardiography and transesophageal echocardiography in the planning and guidance of transcatheter mitral valve therapies. Many of the echo-imaging guidance techniques are applicable to transcatheter intervention as a whole. However, given that the MitraClip is the only device approved for mitral regurgitation at present, specific attention is paid to this procedure, with additional focus on the guidance of noncentral repair. The imaging techniques discussed will be applicable to future devices.

With increasing utilization of cardiac computed tomographic angiography (CTA) and widespread adoption of fusion imaging technology allowing the merger of pre-procedural CTA with fluoroscopy, the ability of CTA to guide structural heart interventions has evolved significantly. It has opened new possibilities in mitral valve (MV) interventions with improved pre-procedural planning and intra-procedural guidance. Given the lack of fluoroscopic landmarks of the mitral apparatus and continued growth of native MV device technologies, the value of CTA will continue to develop. The goal of this chapter is to detail the role of CTA in MV imaging and support for transcatheter therapies.

For patients with paravalvular mitral prosthetic regurgitation, percutaneous repair is an established therapy for the treatment of symptoms of heart failure or hemolytic anemia. Percutaneous repair of paravalvular mitral regurgitation is a complex procedure with unique technical challenges, even when performed in experienced centers. Herein, the author discusses patient selection, catheter-based techniques for repair, and clinical outcomes of percutaneous repair for paravalvular mitral regurgitation.

Targeted transseptal puncture remains the most critical initial part of the overall MitraClip procedure. Care and attention must be implemented for patient safety in choosing the optimal puncture site. A consistent and step-by-step methodical approach is recommended. As experienced operators are targeting more complex and nontraditional pathologic conditions, use of adjunctive tools and maneuvers (outlined in this review) are paramount to achieving successful targeted transseptal access and ultimately procedural success.

Primary mitral regurgitation (MR) owing to degenerative changes in the structural components of the mitral valve is a common acquired valvular pathology in the elderly. Surgical correction with mitral valve repair (MVRe) or replacement (MVR) is the mainstay of therapy. A significant proportion of patients are ineligible for MVRe/MVR owing to prohibitive surgical risk from advanced age, poor ventricular function, or associated comorbidities. Percutaneous mitral valve repair techniques have been developed to fill this void. The edge-to-edge MitraClip has accrued the largest human experience. This paper reviews the available literature on the MitraClip device for treatment of primary MR.

Therapy for mitral regurgitation (MR) has been synonymous with mitral valve surgery. Operative approaches for degenerative MR repair have been associated with excellent results, with durable long term outcomes. Surgery for functional MR has been less successful. MitraClip has shown promise for functional MR, especiall in patinets who are high risk for surgery. The aggregate of non-randomized global experience with MitraClip in functional MR has been consistent in showing improvements in symptoms and left ventricular remodeling. It remains to be seen how MitraClip therapy will compare with best medical therapy. The COAPT trial will clarify this question.

Functional, or secondary, mitral regurgitation (FMR) is clinically important because patient with congestive heart failure with FMR have worse clinical outcomes and associated higher risks than patients without FMR. There is interest in finding repair techniques which may modify the mitral valve dysfunction and reduce the clinical impact. Although several devices have taken advantage of the close anatomical relationship between the coronary sinus and the posterior annulus of the mitral valve, in order to provide a cinching force on the mitral annulus, only the Carillon device is currently in use in humans. A double blind randomized trial is currently being done to evaluate the value of this therapy, building upon the favorable result of three prior safety and efficacy trials, which have led to European approval of the device.

Percutaneous mitral valve therapies are emerging as an alternative option for high-risk patients who are not good candidates for conventional open-heart surgery. Recently, multiple technologies and diversified approaches have been developed and are under clinical study or in preclinical development. This article on transcatheter mitral annuloplasty devices, describes the different technologies, and reports on the initial clinical and preclinical experiences.

Mitral valve disease prevalence is on the rise worldwide, affecting an estimated 2% of the general population. Novel transcatheter mitral valve replacement technologies are being developed and may provide a viable and safe option in patients who are deemed otherwise not suitable candidates for conventional mitral valve surgery. This article reviews these devices and describes trials of first in-human use.

Valve-in-valve and valve-in-ring transcatheter mitral valve replacement can be used in for the treatment of inoperable patients with failing mitral surgical bioprosthesis or valve repairs. Preprocedural multi-image evaluation by a heart team must include transthoracic echocardiogram, transesophageal echocardiogram, and cardiac computed tomography angiography (CTA). CTA is used to determine access site (transapical, transseptal, or transatrial), transcatheter valve size, and landing zone. Though complications can occur (ie, valve embolization, bleeding, or vascular complications), this less invasive procedure has a reported success rate of 70% to 100% and is now increasingly used.

TRANSCATHETER MITRAL VALVE INTERVENTION

THE CLINICS ARE NOW AVAILABLE ONLINE!

Access your subscription at:
www.theclinics.com

PREFACE

A Revolution in Transcatheter Mitral Valve Intervention

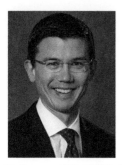

Jason H. Rogers, MD, FACC, FSCAI
Editor

The field of interventional structural heart disease has grown rapidly in the last decade with the introduction of numerous innovations in diagnosis, imaging, and treatment. The initial growth of this new specialty was fueled heavily by the evidence-based commercial approval of transcatheter aortic valve replacement. This therapy has continued to mature and has seen widespread adoption. Interventional therapies for mitral valve disease, and in particular mitral regurgitation, have been slower to develop given the heterogeneity of mitral valve disease states, the anatomic complexity of the mitral valve apparatus, and the challenges of imaging and delivering therapy to the left side of the heart. Despite these challenges, tremendous advances have been made in this field, and although only a few devices have commercial approval at this time, literally dozens of other approaches to mitral valve repair and replacement are under development at various stages of preclinical and early clinical investigation. The clinical need for less invasive therapies for mitral valve disease is undisputed, especially in patients with systolic heart failure and concomitant mitral regurgitation. The fields of interventional cardiology and cardiac surgery are evolving toward utilizing effective transcatheter therapies for mitral valve correction in patients at high surgical risk, with the hope that these technologies will mature to a point where they can be considered a viable alternative therapy in intermediate and lower risk patients.

In this issue of *Interventional Cardiology Clinics*, the reader will find reviews on various topics relevant to transcatheter mitral valve intervention by thought-leaders from around the globe. This issue begins with an excellent article on the normal mitral valve anatomy as well as pathologic disease states. Next, echocardiographic and computed tomographic imaging are covered, followed by procedural and data summaries of mitral paravalvular leak closure, transseptal puncture, and MitraClip therapy for primary and secondary MR. Coronary sinus-based and direct annular approaches to mitral annuloplasty are covered, and the issue concludes with exciting updates on transcatheter mitral valve and valve-in-valve replacement.

Our gratitude goes to the all the contributors to this focus issue, and we hope that you enjoy this unique collection of articles dedicated to the mitral valve revolution.

Jason H. Rogers, MD, FACC, FSCAI
Professor, Cardiovascular Medicine
Director, Interventional Cardiology
University of California, Davis Medical Center
4860 Y Street, Suite 2820
Sacramento, CA 95817, USA

E-mail address:
jhrogers@ucdavis.edu

Intervent Cardiol Clin 5 (2016) ix
http://dx.doi.org/10.1016/j.iccl.2015.10.001
2211-7458/16/$ – see front matter © 2016 Published by Elsevier Inc.

Anatomy and Function of the Normal and Diseased Mitral Apparatus
Implications for Transcatheter Therapy

Elizabeth M. Perpetua, DNP, APRN-BC[a],*,
Dmitry B. Levin, BA[b], Mark Reisman, MD[b]

KEYWORDS

- Mitral valve • Transcatheter valve therapy • Mitral valve apparatus
- Catheter-based intervention

KEY POINTS

- The aortic valve (AV) is anatomically simple and relatively independent of neighboring structures, whereas the mitral valve (MV) apparatus comprises multiple complex structures that must work in synchrony, interdependent with the AV and left ventricle (LV).
- In contrast to AV disease, MV disease is heterogeneous and may result from pathologic changes of any, and often, more than 1, component of the MV apparatus.
- Transcatheter mitral therapy must innovate and expand to address these unique distinctions in MV anatomy, pathoanatomy, disease etiologies, and mechanisms.

 Videos of aortic and subaortic/LVOT flow dynamics accompany this article at http://www. interventional.theclinics.com/

The MV apparatus comprises multiple interdependent structures, actively working in synchrony to open in diastole and close in systole. These characteristics are distinct to the AV, which is the centerpiece of the heart, anatomically simple and relatively independent of neighboring structures, with passive participation in cardiac output. In contrast to AV disease, MV disease is heterogeneous and may result from pathologic changes of any, and often, more than 1, component of the MV apparatus.

Transcatheter mitral therapy subsequently requires an in-depth understanding of the complex MV apparatus (annulus, leaflets, chordae tendinae, and papillary muscle [PM]) and the adjacent structures (left atrium [LA], LV outflow tract [LVOT], AV, coronary sinus, and circumflex artery) (Fig. 1). Various conditions result in pathoanatomical and functional changes of the competent MV. The aim of this review is to describe the anatomy and function of the normal and diseased MV apparatus and the implications for catheter-based intervention.

MITRAL VALVE ANATOMY, PATHOANATOMY, AND FUNCTION
Annulus

The MV lies obliquely in the heart and has a hyperbolic parabolic shape similar to a riding saddle (Fig. 2), with the peaks located at the anterior and posterior horns and the nadir at the commissures. The commissures are distinct triangular segments of tissue that establish continuity between the 2 MV leaflets. Named for the

[a] Division of Cardiothoracic Surgery, Department of Surgery, University of Washington, 1959 Northeast Pacific Street, Box 356171, Seattle, WA 98195, USA; [b] Division of Cardiology, Department of Medicine, University of Washington, 1959 Northeast Pacific Street, Box 356171, Seattle, WA, USA
* Corresponding author.
E-mail address: eperpetu@uw.edu

Intervent Cardiol Clin 5 (2016) 1–16
http://dx.doi.org/10.1016/j.iccl.2015.08.012
2211-7458/16/$ – see front matter © 2016 Elsevier Inc. All rights reserved.

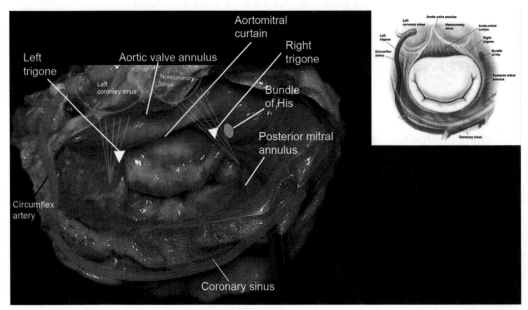

Fig. 1. Comprehensive review of relational anatomy of the MV en face. (*Courtesy of* University of Washington, Seattle, WA; with permission.)

corresponding PMs, the anterolateral commissure (ALC) and posteromedial commissure reinforce a virtual suspension bridge.

The annulus (Fig. 3) separates the LA and the LV and gives attachment to the MV. It is an oval,

or D-shape, in which the anterior annulus is the straight side and the posterior annulus is curved. The anterior annulus composes one-third and the posterior annulus composes two-thirds of the circumference; the medial-lateral diameter

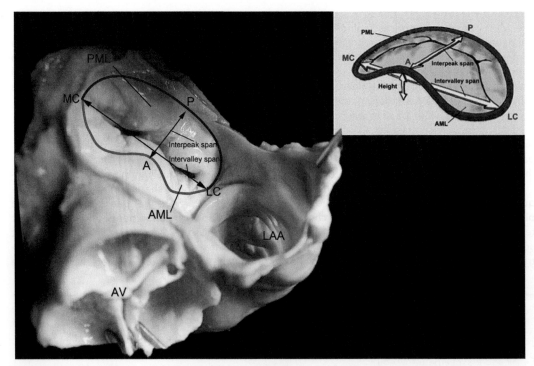

Fig. 2. Hyperbolic parabolic saddle shape of the MV. A, anterior; LC, lateral commissure; MC, medial commissure; P, posterior. (*Courtesy of* University of Washington, Seattle, WA; with permission.)

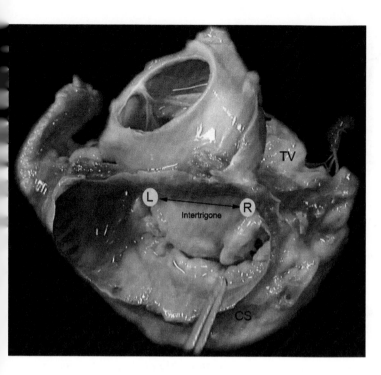

Fig. 3. The MV annulus. The anterior or fibrous annulus is more rigid, owing to the left (L) and right (R) trigones, which are part of the cytoskeleton of the heart. The anterior annulus is exposed to peak tensile forces, whereas the posterior or muscular annulus (forceps) is weaker and more prone to dilatation and calcification. The weakest point of the annulus is at the posterior segment and medial commissural segment, which is where the posterior annulus tends to dilate and fail. (*Courtesy of* University of Washington, Seattle, WA; with permission.)

exceeds the anterior-posterior diameter. The annulus is dynamic, with an area change of 23% to 40% during the cardiac cycle[1]; at midsystole in the normal annulus, the area and perimeter are at their minimum and at their maximum in late diastole.[2,3]

Annulus implies a fibrous ring; however, it is only the anterior annulus that is rigid. The aortic and mitral annuli are anatomically coupled where the AV and the anterior mitral leaflet (AML) are in fibrous continuity, known as the aortomitral curtain by surgeons and the intervalvular fibrosa by echocardiographers.[4] This region is part of the cardiac skeleton; the right and left trigones are the fibrous tissue at the terminal aspects of this continuity.[5] The anterior annulus is subsequently less susceptible to dilatation despite being exposed to peak tensile forces.

The atrioventricular conduction bundle courses through the right fibrous trigone, continuous with the membranous septum, which coupled are referred to as the central fibrous body.[6] The annulus location is variable in relation to adjacent vascular structures but can lie 1 cm below the coronary sinus and 2 cm below the circumflex artery.

The posterior annulus is mostly muscular, with the weakest point at the posterior and medial commissural segments and the posteromedial aspect of the annulus the weakest overall. The posterior annulus is more vulnerable to degenerative changes, such as calcification and dilatation. In conditions that result in LA enlargement, in particular atrial fibrillation, the dilated LA over time may also result in anterior annular dilatation, although typically this is a late finding. Dilation of the annulus transforms its native D-shape or saddle shape into an oval, thereby compromising MV coaptation.

Leaflets

When viewed en face, the D-shaped annulus and the "smile" formed by approximated MV leaflets is well appreciated (**Fig. 4**). The AML is also referred to as the aortic leaflet, and the posterior mitral leaflet (PML) as the mural leaflet, demonstrating their distinct relationships with the AV and the ventricle, respectively. The AML is apical and smooth, tall and narrow; conversely, the PML is short and wide (**Fig. 5**). The PML has a shelf or bracket that inserts into the annulus at the left atrioventricular junction. With LV dilatation, this posterior shelf may be more prominent.

The PML has distinct indentations, readily identifiable by the attachment of primary chords into the body of the leaflet.[7] Distinctly different from a cleft (abnormal recess of leaflet tissue all the way to the annulus), these normal indentations of the PML are referred to as scallops. Starting laterally from the ALC, extending medially to the posteromedial commissure, these

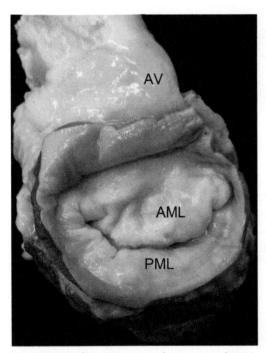

Fig. 4. MV leaflets. (*Courtesy of* University of Washington, Seattle, WA; with permission.)

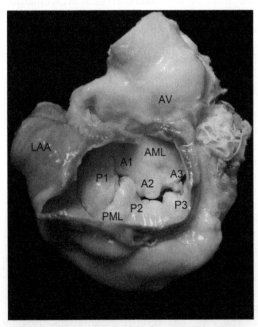

Fig. 5. Overview of the MV, en face view. The AV is superior to and in continuity with the AML. The PML has 3 distinct scallops (P1, P2, and P3), the first (P1) named from the ALC; the AML is divided into 3 segments (A1, A2, and A3) descriptively, without anatomic scallops. At the anterolateral aspect of the MV is the left atrial appendage (LAA). (*Courtesy of* University of Washington, Seattle, WA; with permission.)

scallops are named P1, P2, and P3. The AML has no such indentations; using the reflections of the PML, the AML is similarly labeled A1, A2, and A3 for descriptive purposes.[7]

The leaflets may have a hooded appearance with outpouching toward the LA, observed between chordal attachments.[8] This pocket-like doming is not indicative of prolapse, which is defined by leaflet extension above the plane of the atrioventricular junction (mitral annular plane) during ventricular systole. Primary prolapse is most often due to the floppy valve, in which redundant, thickened leaflet tissue protrudes into the LA.[9] This tissue may be soft and even gelatinous. The PML, particularly at the middle scallop, is most frequently affected, attributed to the annular dilatation of the weaker, muscular posterior annulus. Excessive redundancy and annular dilatation is characteristic of Barlow disease.

Other conditions may result in rigid, nonpliable leaflets. Stiffening of the leaflet tips, along with commissural fusion, is typical of rheumatic heart disease. Morphologic changes due to infective endocarditis also distort and stiffen the MV leaflets. Fibroelastic deficiency, frequently seen in the elderly, may result in less pliable leaflets and chordal rupture.

Clear and rough zones

Two zones exist on the atrial surface of the AML: the peripheral or clear zone and the central or rough zone. The smooth area extending back to the annulus is the clear zone. Named for the nodular surface created by the insertion points of the primary and secondary chordae tendinae, the rough zone is broadest at the lowest or most apical part of the leaflet and narrowest at the commissures. In addition to the rough and clear zones, the PML has a basal zone, where secondary chords from the ventricle insert into the leaflet and separates the clear zone from the annulus.[7] There is also a section of each leaflet that is free of chordal insertion, known as the chord-free zone.

Line of coaptation

The crescentic ridge that separates the rough and clear zones is the line of coaptation. The region extending from the coaptation line to the free edge of the leaflets is the zone of coaptation. This area represents the coaptation surface of the valve, the site where the AML is in contact with the PML when the valve is closed in systole. For normal closure of the MV, the 2 leaflets must align in the same plane in apposition along the single line of coaptation. The depth and length of coaptation are important parameters of MV competency.[7]

Aortomitral Angle and the Cardiac Cycle

Timek and colleagues[10] defined the aortomitral angle (AMA) as the angle between the centroid of the aortic annulus markers, the saddle horn, and the centroid of the mitral annulus markers. This angle may be otherwise described as formed by the intersection of the mitral annulus and the aortic annulus at the intervalvular fibrosa or aortomitral curtain, where the aortic and mitral annuli are coupled.

In systole, the posterior annulus moves towards the apex, while the anterior horn of the saddle moves toward the left atrium. This movement contributes to the late systolic increase of the aortic orifice, and accompanies the aorta in its movement, which increases of the aortomitral angle. In diastole, the anterior horn of the saddle moves up and toward the aortic annulus, which decreases the aortomitral angle, and prepares the MV for the next closure of the AML. The AML participates passively in the mechanism of valve closure. Conversely, the posterior annulus actively contracts: first, the scallops coapt together; then, the PML moves toward the AML, to coordinate closure of the valve.[10]

Chordae Tendinae

There are several sets of fanlike chordae attach to the edge and body of the MV leaflets (Fig. 6). Primary (marginal) chordae insert into the free edge of the leaflet and are responsible for keeping the coaptation zone of the MV in line during systole, preventing prolapse. These thin, delicate chords attach into the free edge of the rough zone, which is the thickest and the toughest aspect of both leaflets. Primary chordae may be further categorized as fan, cleft, or commissural chordae. These delicate chords are the most likely to rupture, particularly posteriorly due to annular or LV dilatation. Cleft chordae divide the leaflets of the PML into scallops. Commissural chordae are critical for maintaining coaptation at the leaflet junctions. At the most medial aspect of the free edge of the leaflets there is typically a chord-free zone.[7]

Secondary chordae insert higher into the body of the MV leaflets at the junction of the rough or clear zone. Strut or stay chords (Fig. 7) are thicker and longer, responsible for maintaining ventricular-valvular continuity, and insert even higher into the basal zone of the leaflet. These chordae are critical to LV geometry, constituting the anatomic interface between the musculature of the LV myocardium at the PMs and the mitral annulus at the fibrous trigones. Sectioning of the anterior stay chords causes an increase in the AMA formed by the aortic and mitral annulus, with the apex of this angle directly connected to the anterior stay chord thorough the aortomitral curtain.[11]

The most reliable way to identify anterior and posterior stay chordae is to locate the most medial of all the basal chordae; the anterior is thicker than the posterior stay chords, suggesting these are under more tension.

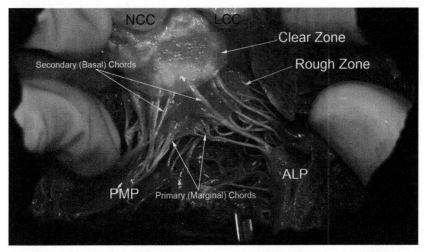

Fig. 6. Overview of chordae tendinae, clear and rough zones. Primary chords insert at the free margin of the leaflets, whereas secondary chords insert higher into the leaflet near the junction of the rough and clear zone. PMP, posteromedial papillary. (*Courtesy of* University of Washington, Seattle, WA; with permission.)

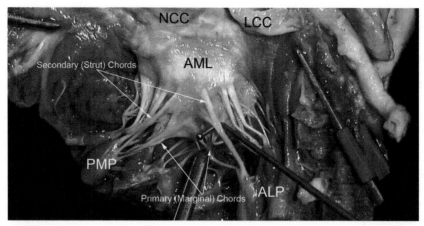

Fig. 7. Stay chordae tendinae. In this image, a strut, stay, or principle chord is isolated; these chordae maintain ventricular-valvular continuity. Anterior stay chordae are under more tension than posterior chordae. ALP, anterolateral papillary; PMP, posteromedial papillary. (*Courtesy of* University of Washington, Seattle, WA; with permission.)

Chordal rupture may be due to tension stress but is often unclear. Various disease states result in primary morphologic changes that may contribute to chordal rupture, such as myxomatous valve disease, fibroelastic deficiency, infective endocarditis, and rheumatic valve disease. Rupture of more than 1 chord rupture causes an acute loss of leaflet support and abrupt onset of loss of coaptation and mitral regurgitation (MR).[12] In these acute cases, the LA is of normal size and the heart function is typically normal. Conversely, progressive or chronic loss of MV coaptation due to annular, leaflet, or chordal abnormalities is usually accompanied by LA enlargement and subsequent changes to other interdependent structures and their function.

Papillary Muscles and the Left Ventricle
The PMs are the muscular component of the MV apparatus. Each PM gives rise to chords that insert into both leaflets on its respective side (**Fig. 8**) and insert into the ventricle at the middle and apical third. If aptly named for the attitudinally correct location, the anterolateral PM would be labeled superior and the posteromedial PM inferior (**Fig. 9**).

The anterolateral PM originates between the lateral and inferolateral LV wall and gives rise

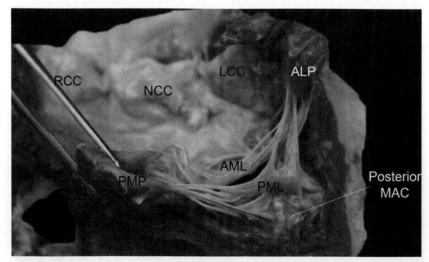

Fig. 8. PMs supply chordae tendinae to each mitral leaflet on its respective side. This image also demonstrates the relationship of the AV and AML, the aortomitral curtain, and shows calcium between the left coronary cusp (LCC), and noncoronary cusp (NCC). There is LVOT calcium as well as posterior MAC. ALP, anterolateral papillary; PMP, posteromedial papillary; RCC, right coronary cusp of the aortic valve. (*Courtesy of* University of Washington, Seattle, WA; with permission.)

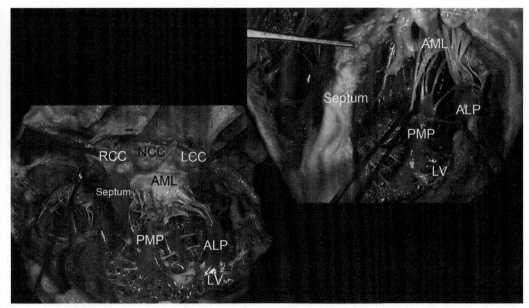

Fig. 9. Insertion of chordae tendinae into PM heads and PM body into the LV. PM bodies insert into the middle and apical third of the LV. ALP, anterolateral papillary; PMP, posteromedial papillary; RCC, right coronary cusp of the aortic valve. (*Courtesy of* University of Washington, Seattle, WA; with permission.)

to the chords that attach to the most lateral and central part of the MV (A1, A2, P1, and P2). The posteromedial PM is located at the most inferior wall of the LV and gives rise to the chords that attach to the most medial and central part of the MV (A2, A3, P2, and P3).[13] Anatomic variations of this configuration may be observed. Often times, several smaller muscle heads replace the single posteromedial PM. Another anomalous example is depicted in **Fig. 10** demonstrating the anteromedial PM inserting directly into the AML.

To brace the leaflets and chordae for the abrupt rise in intraventricular pressure, the PM contracts before the LV wall. This is followed by synchronous contraction of the PM and LV, which supports the chords and prevents the overshooting of the MV leaflets in systole.[14]

It must be recognized that these structures are dependent on adequate myocardial blood flow through the coronary arteries for optimal function. The anterolateral PM is often a single structure with dual blood supply from the left coronary artery, whereas the posteromedial PM

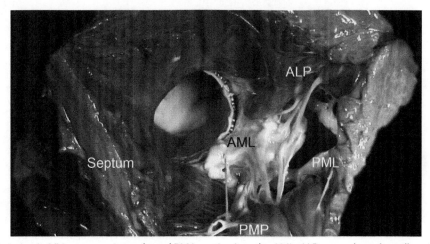

Fig. 10. Variation in MV anatomy. Anterolateral PM insertion into the AML. ALP, anterolateral papillary; PMP, posteromedial papillary. (*Courtesy of* University of Washington, Seattle, WA; with permission.)

is usually a multihead structure with blood supply from only the right coronary artery.

These subvalvular structures may contribute to valve incompetence in the presence of ischemia due to ischemia or PM rupture due to acute myocardial infarction. Dysfunction of the PM may be classified according to the continuity with the LV.[15] The loss of PM and LV continuity is due to trauma or infarct, resulting in acute incompetence of the MV and MR. Dysfunction without loss in PM and LV continuity is due to (1) ischemia without infarct and is often highly acute and episodic, mild or severe, and (2) infarct, which results in ischemic cardiomyopathy and chronic incompetence of the MV. Changes in LV geometry, such as LV dilatation with remodeling, also have an impact on MV coaptation.

Left Ventricular Outflow Tract

The LVOT is the region of the LV that lies between the ventricular septum and the AML. It is a subvalvular ring (Fig. 11) comprising the outlet muscular septum, membranous septum, anterior LV free wall, and anterior MV leaflet.[16] Anteriorly the LVOT comprises the membranous and the muscular septum. The membranous septum is contiguous with the right lateral wall of the aortic root, the medial wall of the right atrium, and a small part of the septal leaflet of the tricuspid valve. The muscular septum is smooth walled and at its junction with the membranous septum lies the atrioventricular bundle. The posterior wall of the LVOT is formed by the LV free wall, or intervalvar septum, and the AML.

The AML is an important component of flow through the LVOT. Abnormal forward motion of the AML during systole causes LVOT obstruction,[17] which may occur in the absence of asymmetric septal hypertrophy, previously known as idiopathic subaortic stenosis, which narrows the LVOT at the onset of systole.[18] The coupling of the aortic and mitral annuli and the relationship of the AML to the LVOT have an impact on the flow of blood through the AV and cardiac output.

MITRAL VALVE DISEASE

MV pathoanatomy and disease are complex and heterogeneous. Additionally, multiple lesions and mixed valve disease may be present in an individual patient. In-depth understanding of the disease mechanisms is key to therapy selection.

MR is the most common valve lesion worldwide.[19,20] Heterogeneous changes in MV and LV morphology result in incompetent leaflet closure and systolic regurgitation of blood into the LA, thereby compromising LV pressure and forward flow. The underlying etiology of MR is classified as predominantly primary (degenerative or organic) or secondary (functional).[21,22] Carpentier and colleagues' classification of MR

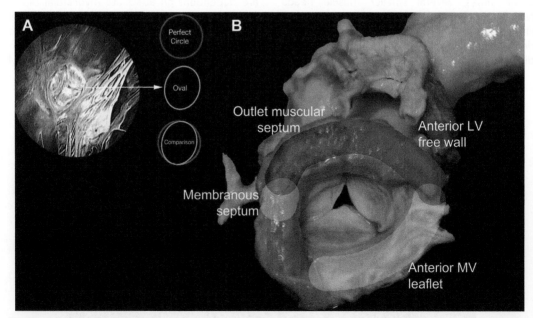

Fig. 11. (A) The LVOT is an oval with dynamic changes throughout the cardiac cycle. (B) Subvalvar LVOT ring comprises the anterior LV free wall, anterior MV leaflet, membranous septum, and outlet muscular septum. (Courtesy of University of Washington, Seattle, WA; with permission.)

(Fig. 12) describes 3 major classes dysfunction of leaflet motion. This taxonomy assists in defining the mechanism of MR and thereby planning catheter-based interventions.

Primary MR is due to 1 or more of the MV components preventing normal leaflet coaptation. Myxomatous MV disease, MV prolapse or flail leaflet, chordal rupture, rheumatic heart disease, fibroelastic deficiency, and endocarditis are some of the conditions that may result in primary MR. Surgical repair or replacement, or transcatheter repair for patients who have high or excessive surgical risk, is recommended for severe primary MR.[21]

In secondary MR, the MV leaflets are structurally normal, but coaptation is compromised due to tethering or restriction of leaflet motion due to dilatation of the LV, MV annulus, or LA. Treatment consists of guideline-directed medical therapy, cardiac resynchronization therapy, and, if warranted, coronary artery revascularization.[21]

Mitral stenosis (MS) is the diastolic narrowing of the MV orifice, typically due to calcification of the MV leaflets or annulus seen in the elderly or those with a history of radiation heart disease or rheumatic commissural fusion, particularly in areas where antibiotics are not dispensed.[20] Percutaneous balloon commissurotomy is an evidence-based treatment of rheumatic MS[2]; however, options for treating MS due to calcified MV stenosis are limited. Often calcified MS occurs with concomitant MR, and the burden and location of calcification pose significant challenges for treatment.

MV disease, namely MR with congestive heart failure, carries a 1-year mortality of up to 50% in symptomatic patients.[23–25] The standard of care is surgical MV repair or replacement[21]; however, up to 40% of patients do not undergo MV surgery.[19] Catheter-based therapy has emerged to address this undertreated patient population.

IMPLICATIONS FOR TRANSCATHETER MITRAL VALVE THERAPY

In the new era of transcatheter valve therapy, comprehensive understanding of the myriad etiologies of MV disease is critical. There may be multiple mechanisms, and identifying the culprit mechanism(s) requires precise assessment for procedural selection and planning.[28] The pathoanatomy of each component of the MV apparatus and their interdependent relationships carry specific implications for catheter-based intervention.

Anatomic Target
Annulus
Annuloplasty of the MV has been targeted in both surgical and catheter-based intervention with varying levels of success. The

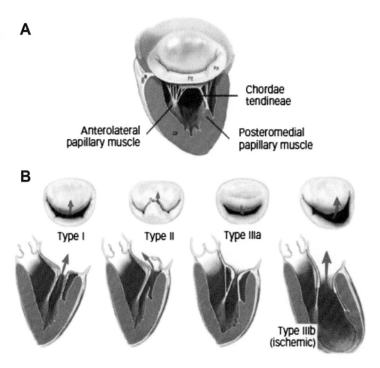

A

Anterolateral papillary muscle

Chordae tendineae

Posteromedial papillary muscle

B

Type I   Type II   Type IIIa

Type IIIb (ischemic)

Fig. 12. The Carpentier classification of MR. (A) Normal MV anatomy. (B) Types of MR. Type I, normal leaflet motion (annular dilatation, leaflet perforation, or clefts). Type II, excessive leaflet motion (chordal rupture, flail). Type III, restricted leaflet motion. Type IIIa, restricted leaflet motion greater in diastole than systole (rheumatic MV disease). Type IIIb, restricted leaflet motion greater in systole due to leaflet tethering secondary to LV dilatation and remodeling (infarct).

hyperparabolic paraboloid shape and dynamic nature of the annulus are complex qualities to incorporate in the development of a conformational device (Fig. 13).

Annular area is also an important consideration. The normal MV annular area is the largest of the heart valves, and dilatation of the LA or LV, as seen in functional MR, further increases annular dimensions. Annular diameter may exceed 45 mm from commissure to commissure. Devices must subsequently span a larger range of sizes, and their specifications must meet the challenge of remaining consistent across multiple, larger sizes. Also, devices that seek to approximate the leaflets of an MV with a severely dilated annulus must also consider what may be an expansive gap required for leaflet approximation.

The muscular posterior annulus is not only prone to dilatation but also to mitral annular calcification (MAC) (Fig. 14). Annular rigidity from severe MAC may impair devices that target annular reduction via a supra-annular, infra-annular, or coronary sinus approach. Moreover, severe MAC may actually reduce annular dimensions and carry an associated diastolic inflow gradient. Thus, assessment of MAC and MS severity is crucial for devices that reduce the MV area (MVA) or orifice dimensions, which may further decrease the MVA or mean pressure gradient.

Leaflets

Leaflet anatomy and pathoanatomy is a primary consideration for devices that restore leaflet coaptation by approximating the leaflet tissue. For these devices, favorable primary MR anatomy/pathoanatomy includes P2 prolapse and some bileaflet prolapse.[26]

Other primary leaflet pathology carries specific challenges. Flail leaflet can make leaflet grasping or capture difficult. Excessive leaflet redundancy presents challenges to achieving coaptation along a single line, resulting in multiple jets of MR; thus, devices aimed at approximating the leaflets may displace, more so than reduce, MR. Leaflet calcification may render the leaflet more fragile and at higher risk for perforation.

Normal leaflet anatomy seen in functional MR is generally favorable, except if the leaflets are too restricted or tethered, typically seen with the posterior leaflet due to LV dilatation. The posterior leaflet may actually be nearly vertical and difficult for devices to grasp or retain the leaflet tissue.

Aortomitral continuity, aortomitral angle, and the left ventricular outflow tract

Transcatheter mitral therapies must respect the aortomitral continuity, AMA, and LVOT to prevent LVOT obstruction. Annuloplasty devices must note the coupling of the aortic and mitral annuli at the aortomitral curtain, whereas catheter-based therapies, in particular transcatheter MV implants, may shift the AML or reduce the size of the LVOT.

Calculation of the AMA is key to understanding the LVOT interaction and the impact on this by transcatheter mitral therapies (Fig. 15). A

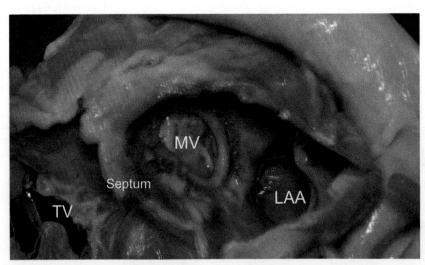

Fig. 13. Hyperparabolic paraboloid mitral annulus: shape and dynamism of the annulus presents unique challenges to transcatheter MV intervention. D-shaped surgical mitral annuloplasty ring is shown. (*Courtesy of* University of Washington, Seattle, WA; with permission.)

A

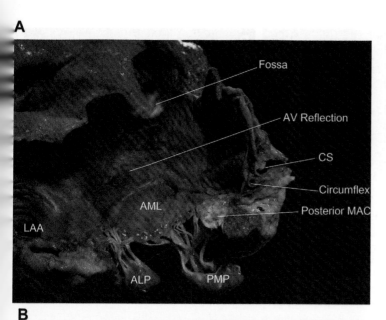

Fig. 14. Calcification of the MV apparatus: location, severity, and distribution of calcium may involve several structures of the MV complex and must be carefully considered in MV intervention. (A) Severe MAC and calcified leaflets may increase risk of annular or leaflet perforation. (B) Severe posterior MAC may increase risk of paravalvular insufficiency. (C) Calcification of the MV complex may contribute to a decreased MV area and increase the diastolic inflow gradient. The baseline assessment is a critical for catheter-based intervention that may exacerbate MS. ALP, anterolateral papillary; PMP, posteromedial papillary. (Courtesy of University of Washington, Seattle, WA; with permission.)

B

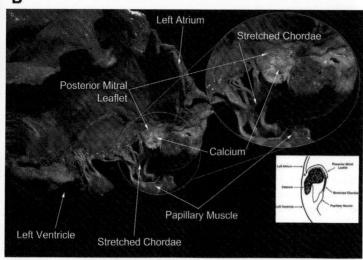

C

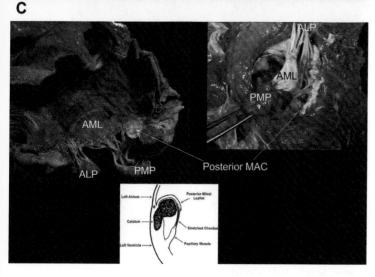

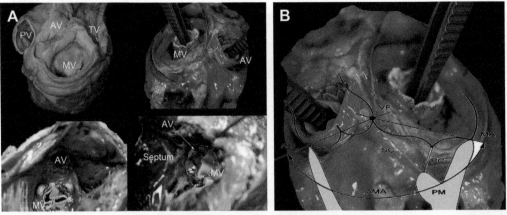

Fig. 15. AMA and LVOT/sub-LVOT relationship. (A) Respecting the AMA is key to understanding the interaction of the LVOT. A new LVOT, or neo-LVOT, may be constructed by transcatheter MV devices. PV, pulmonary vein. (B) Forceps midorifice of the aortic and MVs represent the trajectory and, in this example, create an obtuse angle. IVF, intervalvular fibrosa; MA, mitral annulus; PC, primary chords; PM, papillary muscle; SC, strut chords. (Courtesy of University of Washington, Seattle, WA; with permission.)

new or neo-LVOT may be created with these devices, particularly in transcatheter MV implantation. As previously described, the risk of LVOT obstruction increases the more acute the angle; conversely, the risk of LVOT obstruction decreases the more obtuse the angle. Knowledge of an acute AMA in the preplanning stage may exclude the use of certain catheter-based interventions.

The concern for systolic anterior motion of the MV and LVOT obstruction is a historical concern from the surgical literature. In surgical MV repair or replacement, obstruction of the LVOT occurs when the mitral coaptation line is displaced anteriorly. The AML is a component of flow in the AV (Fig. 16, Videos 1 and 2) and must be respected by all devices. The predisposition for systolic anterior motion is associated with a small baseline LVOT, asymmetric septal hypertrophy, and a small ventricle. Many of these findings may occur together in an individual patient.[27,28] The anterior leaflet length and compliance, as well as depth of implant and size, all have an impact on the interaction with the LVOT.

Subvalvar apparatus

The subvalvular apparatus is targeted by interventions that seek to repair the chords. Surgical

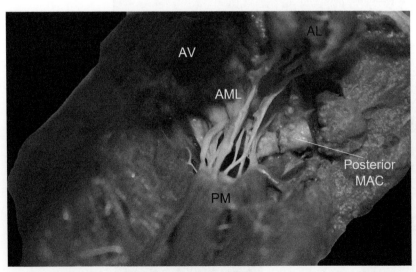

Fig. 16. Unique relationship of the AML and the LVOT: the AML is a component of flow in the AV. AL, anterolateral. (Courtesy of University of Washington, Seattle, WA; with permission.)

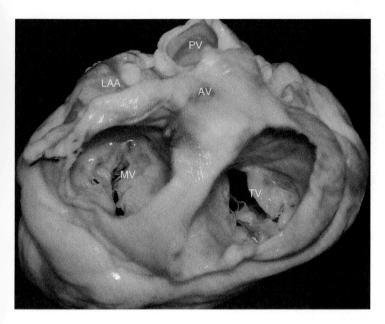

Fig. 17. Transseptal approach for catheter-based mitral therapies: orientation for transseptal puncture is critical and must consider the attitudinally correct anatomic position of the MV, seen here en face. PV, pulmonary vein. (*Courtesy of* University of Washington, Seattle, WA; with permission.)

strategies have included securing new synthetic chordae tendinae into the leaflet and PM. Catheter-based devices may use a similar strategy. Pathoanatomy of the subvalvular apparatus, including ruptured chordae, calcified chordae, and ischemic or infarcted PM, must be considered when determining whether transcatheter chordal repair is favorable.

Access for Therapy
Transseptal approach
Successful transseptal puncture for catheter-based mitral intervention requires extensive knowledge of relational anatomy of the MV (Figs. 17 and 18). Puncture of the fossa ovalis is complex, because its relationship to the MV is not fixed. With MR or MS, the LA may dilated and the fossa may be larger, or the interatrial septum may be hostile due to bowing of and sliding off the fossa secondary to fluid volume overload. Assessment of the interatrial septum for septal defects is key; although seemingly convenient, defects, such as a patent foramen ovale, must be avoided for entry into the LA due its anterior orientation. Traversing the septum through the patent foramen ovale creates disadvantageous anterior and superior orientation. Overall, a superior and posterior entry increases the likelihood of adequate height over the MV to allow for maneuvering and positioning for successful intervention.

Transapical approach
Experience with transapical access is from transcatheter AV replacement (TAVR) (Fig. 19); these

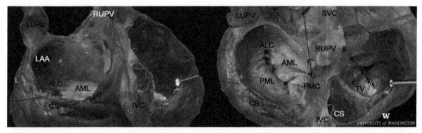

Fig. 18. Transseptal approach for catheter-based mitral therapies: understanding the comprehensive, unique relationships of the MV with adjacent structures is necessary for optimal transseptal puncture. CS, coronary sinus; IVC, inferior vena cava; LAA, left atrial appendage; LUPV, left upper pulmonary vein; RUPV, right upper pulmonary vein; SVC, superior vena cava; TV; tricuspid valve. (*Courtesy of* University of Washington, Seattle, WA; with permission.)

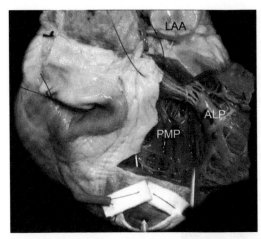

Fig. 19. Transapical access and closure presents different challenges in transcatheter MV therapy compared with TAVR. Compensatory mechanisms for AS result in LV hypertrophy, whereas for MR, the result is LV remodeling with dilatation and thinning. Transcatheter MVs are also larger than those used for TAVR, requiring a larger sheath in an LV that may be more likely to be dilated and thinned. These are important considerations for complications due to bleeding and difficulty with apical closure. ALP, anterolateral papillary; PMP, posteromedial papillary. (*Courtesy of* University of Washington, Seattle, WA; with permission.)

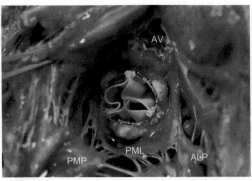

Fig. 21. Transapical approach for catheter-based mitral therapies: preservation of the subvalvular apparatus is paramount, particularly during apical access and transcatheter MV device deployment. ALP, anterolateral papillary; PMP, posteromedial papillary. (*Courtesy of* University of Washington, Seattle, WA; with permission.)

ventricles tend to be hypertrophied, whereas the LV with MV disease, especially MR, may be thin, dilated, and at times compromised with ischemic or nonviable infarct. With MR, the function of the LV is also often compromised and the apex may be aneurysmal or contain thrombus. The MV, as previously described, is also the largest of the heart valves; thus, devices generally require a larger sheath than is used with TAVR. A larger sheath accessing a dilated, thin LV apex may pose increased risk of bleeding complications and difficulty with apical closure. Moreover, avoidance of the subvalvar apparatus is paramount while advancing devices (Fig. 20), to prevent injury to critical structures (Fig. 21). The LV must be comprehensively assessed to determine whether the apex is amenable not only for access but also for closure.

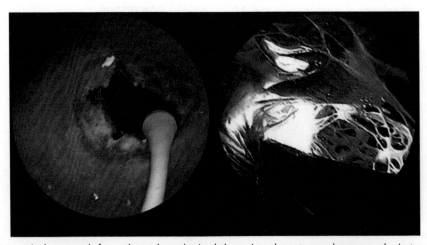

Fig. 20. Transapical approach for catheter-based mitral therapies: the retrograde approach via transapical access requires fastidious attention to the mitral subvalvar apparatus to prevent injury to PMs and chordae tendineae while advancing devices from the apex. (*Courtesy of* University of Washington, Seattle, WA; with permission.)

SUMMARY

The MV apparatus comprises multiple complex structures that must work in synchrony, interdependent with the AV and LV. In contrast, the AV is anatomically simple and relatively independent of neighboring structures. As described, MV disease is heterogeneous and may result from pathologic changes of any, and often, more than 1, component of the MV apparatus. These unique distinctions in MV anatomy, pathoanatomy, disease etiologies, and mechanisms provide tremendous opportunity for innovation and advances in the field of transcatheter mitral therapy.

SUPPLEMENTARY DATA

Videos related to this article can be found online at http://dx.doi.org/10.1016/j.iccl.2015.08.012.

REFERENCES

1. Ormiston JA, Shah PM, Tei C, et al. Size and motion of the mitral valve annulus in man. I. A two-dimensional echocardiographic method and findings in normal subjects. Circulation 1981;64:113–20.
2. Davis PK, Kinmouth JB. The movements of the annulus of the mitral valve. J Cardiovasc Surg 1963;4:427.
3. Flachskampf FA, Chandra S, Gaddipatti A, et al. Analysis of shape and motion of the mitral annulus with and without cardiomyopathy by echocardiographic 3-dimensional reconstruction. J Am Soc Echocardiogr 2000;13:277–87.
4. Yacoub MH, Kilner PJ, Birks EJ, et al. The aortic outflow and root: a tale of dynamism and crosstalk. Ann Thorac Surg 1999;68:S37–43.
5. Berdajs D, Zund G, Camenisch C, et al. Annulus fibrosus of the mitral valve: reality or myth. J Cardiovasc Surg 2007;22:406–9.
6. Ho S. Anatomy of the mitral valve. Heart 2002; 88(Suppl IV):iv5–10.
7. Ranganathan N, Lam JHC, Wigle ED, et al. Morphology of the human mitral valve II. The valve leaflets. Circulation 1970;41:459–67.
8. Becker AE, de Wit APM. The mitral valve apparatus: a spectrum of normality relevant to mitral valve prolapse. Br Heart J 1980;42:680–9.
9. Davies MJ, Moore BP, Braimbridge MV. The floppy mitral valve. Study of incidence, pathology, and complications in surgical, necropsy, and forensic material. Br Heart J 1978;40:468–81.
10. Timek TA, Green GR, Tibayan FA, et al. Aortomitral annular dynamics. Ann Thorac Surg 2003; 76:1944–50.
11. Xiong F, Yeo JH, Chong CK, et al. Transsection of anterior basal stay chords alters left ventricular outflow dynamics and wall shear stress. J Heart Valve Dis 2008;17:54–61.
12. Ronan JA, Steelman RB, DeLeon AC, et al. The clinical diagnosis of acute severe MR. Am J Cardiol 1971;284:37.
13. Rusted IE, Shiefley CH, Edwards JE. Studies of the mitral valve I. Anatomic features of the normal mitral valve and associated structures. Circulation 1952;6:825–31.
14. Roberts WC, Cohen LS. Left ventricular papillary muscles. Description of the normal and a survey of conditions causing them to be abnormal. Circulation 1972;46:138–54.
15. Mitall AK, Langston M, Cohn KE, et al. Combined papillary muscle and LV wall dysfunction as a cause of MR. Circulation 1971;44:174.
16. Walmsley R. Anatomy of left ventricular outflow tract. Br Heart J 1979;41:263–7.
17. Henry WL, Clark CE, Griffith JM, et al. Mechanism of left ventricular outflow tract obstruction in patients with obstructive asymmetrical septal hypertrophy (idiopathic hypertrophic subaortic stenosis). Am J Cardiol 1975;35:337–45.
18. Crawford MH, Groves BM, Horwitz LD. Dynamic left ventricular outflow tract obstruction and systolic anterior motion of the mitral valve in the absence of asymmetrical septal hypertrophy. Am J Med 1978;65:703–8.
19. Iung B, Baron G, Butchrat EG, et al. A prospective surgey of patients with valvular heart disease in Europe: the Euro Heart Survey on valvular heart disease. Eur Heart J 2003;24:1231–43.
20. Nkomo V, Gardin J, Skelton T, et al. Burden of valvular heart diseases: a population-based study. Lancet 2006;368:1005–11.
21. Nishimura RA, Otto CM, Bonow RO, et al. 2014 AHA/ACC guideline for the management of patients with valvular heart disease: executive summary: a report of the American College of Cardiology/American Heart Association Task Force on practice guidelines. J Am Coll Cardiol 2014;63: 2438–88.
22. Carpentier A, Adams DH, Filsoufi F. Carpentier's reconstructive valve surgery. From valve analysis to valve reconstruction. Philadelphia: Saunders, Elsevier; 2010.
23. Cioffi G, Tarantini L, DeFeo S, et al. Functional mitral regurgitation predicts 1-year mortality in elderly patients with systolic chronic heart failure. Eur J Heart Fail 2005;7:1112–7.
24. Grigoni F, Tribouilloy C, Avierinos JF, et al, MIDA Investigators. Outcomes in mitral regurgitation due to flail leaflets a multicenter European study. JACC Cardiovasc Imaging 2008;1: 133–41.

25. Enriquez-Sarano M, Avierinos JF, Messika-Zeitoun D, et al. Quantitative determinants of the outcome of asymptomatic mitral regurgitation. N Engl J Med 2005;352:857–83.

26. Tamburino C, Ussia G, Maisano F, et al. Percutaneous mitral valve repair with the MitraClip system: acute results from a real world setting. Eur Heart J 2010;31:1382–9.

27. Lee KS, Stewart WJ, Lever HM, et al. Mechanism of outflow tract obstruction causing failed mitral valve repair: anterior displacement of leaflet coaptation. Circulation 1993;88(5 Pt 2):1124–9.

28. Maisano F, Buzzatti N, Taramasso M, et al. Mitral transcatheter technologies. Rambam Maimonides Med J 2013;4:e0015.

Echocardiographic Imaging of the Mitral Valve for Transcatheter Edge-to-Edge Repair

Jeffrey M. Paulsen, MD, Thomas W. Smith, MD*

KEYWORDS

- 3D Transesophageal echocardiography • Procedural guidance
- Percutaneous mitral valve repair • MitraClip

KEY POINTS

- Advances in echocardiography have paralleled advances in percutaneous mitral valve repair, resulting in the ability to guide less invasive procedures more accurately and seamlessly.
- MitraClip mitral valve repair requires unique imaging approaches to successfully treat noncentral primary valve disorder.
- The echocardiographer must anticipate how each planned clip will affect the leaflet morphology around the clip.
- Each clip placement will affect the ability and success of the subsequent clip placement.

INTRODUCTION

Echocardiography continues to be the most effective imaging tool for the diagnosis and follow-up of mitral valve disease. The diagnosis of mitral regurgitation (MR) or stenosis is generally accomplished with the use of transthoracic imaging, whereas transesophageal imaging, given the posterior probe location, is ideally positioned for clear resolution of mitral valve structure, which is critically important in understanding the underlying etiology of mitral valve disease and for management and procedural planning. With the development of transcatheter intervention for the mitral valve and other structures, there has been a coevolution in echocardiography. True to the adage of necessity being the mother of invention, the milieu of echo imaging has expanded to real-time support and guidance of structural intervention. In this role, early adopters have recognized the value but also the limitations of 2-dimensional (2D)

imaging. Real-time 3-dimensional (3D) imaging developed in the context of 2D limitations. The advantages of 3D imaging in mitral valve diagnosis and intervention are many, with the clearest example being the ability to obtain en-face views of the valve (visualization of the entire atrial aspect of the valve and adjacent structures in one real-time view). With a more intuitive anatomic presentation, this 3D modality facilitates direct communication with the interventional team, both before and during the procedure, in a graphical representation that all members of the team can interpret and discuss. Consequently, 2D and 3D transesophageal echocardiography (TEE) is now indispensable in mitral valve transcatheter intervention.

This review addresses the use of transthoracic echocardiography (TTE) and TEE in the planning and guidance of transcatheter mitral valve therapies. Many of the echo-imaging guidance techniques are applicable to transcatheter intervention as a whole. However, given that the

---

Division of Cardiovascular Medicine, Department of Internal Medicine, University of California Davis Health System, Sacramento, CA 95817, USA
* Corresponding author. UC Davis Medical Center, 4860 Y Street, Suite 2820, Sacramento, CA 95817.
E-mail address: twrsmith@ucdavis.edu

MitraClip (Abbott Vascular, Santa Clara, CA) is the only device approved by the Food and Drug Administration (FDA) for MR at present, specific attention is paid to this procedure, with additional focus on the guidance of noncentral repair. The imaging techniques discussed will be applicable to future devices.

EVALUATION OF MITRAL VALVE REGURGITATION WITH ECHOCARDIOGRAPHY

Evaluation of chronic MR is nuanced, given that the distinction between primary versus secondary MR has significant implications for management strategy.

In general, clinical assessment and TTE provide most of the useful data for evaluating the severity of MR and initial clinical decision-making. Particularly with secondary (functional) MR, in addition to the finding of significant MR, the expectation is to define left ventricular structural abnormalities on the echocardiogram, including depressed left ventricular systolic function, left ventricular and/or atrial chamber dilatation, and Doppler evidence of elevated intracardiac pressures. By contrast, primary (degenerative) MR involves abnormality of one or more of the components of the valve apparatus (leaflets, chordae tendineae, papillary muscles, annulus).[1]

Consistent with this discussion, pre-MitraClip evaluation begins with TTE for confirmation of MR severity. A thorough 2D structural assessment should be performed for chamber enlargement, wall motion abnormalities, and gross valve derangements such as perforation, flail leaflet, leaflet tethering, and mal-coaptation, among others. Doppler and color flow interrogation of the mitral valve and pulmonary veins allows for thorough quantitative and qualitative assessment of the severity of valve disease. Based on the updated 2014 American College of Cardiology/American Heart Association Valvular Heart Disease Guidelines, there are now separate criteria for valve severity depending on pathology (primary vs secondary MR) (Tables 1 and 2). MR classification for severe secondary MR occurs at lower Doppler thresholds than primary MR.[1]

At present, the FDA indication for MitraClip is for treatment of moderate to severe ($\geq$3+) primary MR in patients who have been evaluated as appropriate by a heart team and deemed to be at prohibitive risk for mitral valve surgery.

Given the improved image resolution of the mitral valve, all patients being evaluated for MitraClip routinely undergo TEE to determine valve abnormality and assess whether the morphology of the affected valve is suitable for percutaneous repair. During the initial EVEREST trials, intervention was limited to A2-P2 area,

Table 1 Severity classification of primary MR		
Grade	Definition	Valve Hemodynamics
A	At risk of MR	No MR jet or small central jet area <20% LA on Doppler Small vena contracta
B	Progressive MR	Central jet MR 20%–40% LA or late systolic eccentric jet MR Vena contracta <0.7 cm Regurgitant volume <60 mL Regurgitant fraction <50% ERO <0.40 cm^2 Angiographic grade 1–2+
C	Asymptomatic severe MR	Central jet MR >40% LA or holosystolic eccentric jet MR Vena contracta $\geq$0.7 cm Regurgitant volume $\geq$60 mL Regurgitant fraction $\geq$50% ERO $\geq$0.40 cm^2 Angiographic grade 3–4+

D	Symptomatic severe MR	Same as grade C, with the following clinical findings:
		    Decreased exercise tolerance
		    Exertional dyspnea

Abbreviations: ERO, effective regurgitant orifice area; LA, left atrium; MR, mitral regurgitation.

Adapted from Nishimura RA, Otto CM, Bonow RO, et al. 2014 AHA/ACC guideline for the management of patients with valvular heart disease: a report of the American College of Cardiology/American Heart Association Task Force on Practice Guidelines. J Am Coll Cardiol 2014;63:e57–185; with permission.

Table 2
Severity classification of secondary MR

Grade	Definition	Valve Hemodynamics
A	At risk of MR	No MR jet or small central jet area <20% LA on Doppler Small vena contracta <0.30 cm
B	Progressive MR	ERO <0.20 cm² Regurgitant volume <30 mL Regurgitant fraction <50%
C	Asymptomatic severe MR	ERO ≥0.20 cm² Regurgitant volume ≥30 mL Regurgitant fraction ≥50%

D	Symptomatic severe MR	Same as grade C, with the following clinical findings:
		  Heart failure symptoms due to MR despite revascularization
		    and optimization of medical therapy
		  Decreased exercise tolerance
		  Exertional dyspnea

Adapted from Nishimura RA, Otto CM, Bonow RO, et al. 2014 AHA/ACC guideline for the management of patients with valvular heart disease: a report of the American College of Cardiology/American Heart Association Task Force on Practice Guidelines. J Am Coll Cardiol 2014;63:e57–185; with permission.

with predominantly central jets.[2] These inclusion criteria were certainly relevant in the early evaluation of MitraClip and were part of the EVEREST II trial. Of patients randomized to MitraClip in EVEREST II, 73% had primary disease.[3] In commercial use, a greater number of clinical cases are now targeting noncentral deployment targets. Consequently, an additional burden has fallen on TEE to outline the complexities of valve lesions and guide procedural success. With additional imaging techniques, non–A2-P2 MR may be successfully treated.[4]

TRANSESOPHAGEAL ECHOCARDIOGRAPHY PROCEDURE
Image Optimization
As a general comment on valve visualization, echocardiographic image quality is optimized when beam transmission occurs through low-density structures. Mitral valve image acquisition for valve assessment and procedural guidance is primarily performed in the mid-esophageal position, with the TEE probe head essentially parallel to the valve plane and the ultrasound beam transmitting through the long axis of the left atrium (ie, with no intervening structures between the posterior left atrial wall and the valve). The probe may need to be higher in the esophagus and significantly retro-flexed to attain a parallel probe position, especially in more vertical hearts (**Fig. 1**).

Building the Mitral Valve Image
When screening before and imaging during an intervention, the echocardiographer must develop a complete understanding of the valve

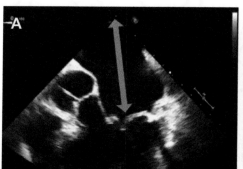
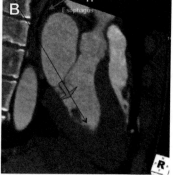

Fig. 1. (*A*) Optimal echo transmission from posterior left atrial wall to the mitral valve (*double arrow*): imaging through soft tissue can lead to image degradation. (*B*) Computed tomography (CT) image of mitral valve demonstrating a very vertical LV (*large arrow*) requiring significant retroflexion of the TEE probe to optimally image the mitral valve (esophagus, *small arrow*).

anatomy from both 2D and 3D perspectives. These images must then be displayed in a manner that all team members can follow. This knowledge and skill is imperative for assessment of the likelihood of success, intervention planning, and, ultimately, real-time guidance.

From the mid-esophageal view, with the omniplane at 0°, the A2-P2 segments should be seen in the 4-chamber view. From this initial position, the remaining segments of the valve may be visualized. Although most mitral valve TEEs are performed with predefined omniplane angles (typically 0°, 30°, 60°, 90°, 120°, and 140°), the authors prefer a more continuous method of imaging, similar to that described by Foster and colleagues.[5] Essentially, the authors sweep and image at 3 different omniplanes defined by the mitral anatomy. The first image begins at 0°, where the probe is withdrawn so that the lateral annulus (adjacent to the left atrial appendage [LAA]) is visualized; the probe is then advanced in the esophagus from lateral to medial, ending at the medial annulus (Fig. 2A). The next images are obtained with the imaging plane that shows the major axis of the valve, the bicommissural view, which typically is between 45° and 70° and demonstrates the P1-A2-P3 scallops. The probe is then rotated clockwise for visualization of A1-A2-A3 and then counterclockwise to P1-P2-P3 (Fig. 2B). Finally, at approximately 120° to 140° (minor axis of the valve), the left ventricular outflow tract is seen, with an adjacent mitral view of A2-P2. This plane optimizes visualization of central valve coaptation for measurement of flail width/gap. At this angle, clockwise rotation of the probe sweeps medially to the medial commissure and counterclockwise to the lateral commissure. This view has been the standard grasping view for MitraClip deployment, as A2-P2 was the traditional central position for clip placement because it provides a perpendicular imaging plane to the mitral valve line of coaptation (Fig. 2C). With a lateral or medial scallop grasp, the omniplane angle may vary considerably (see later discussion).

The authors favor Foster's method for assessing the mitral valve. Although imaging to standardized angles with stereotypical imaging planes has been recommended in the early literature, the authors find that the continuous method of sweeping through the valve offers a more complete understanding of the valve morphology. This method allows for visualization and understanding of the entirety of the valve instead of making assumptions about the morphology in the gaps between stereotypical image planes. This approach is similar to looking at a large object in the dark with a narrow-beam flashlight. If you only shine the light at predetermined spots, you will not see the whole object. If you sweep the light back and forth, you will visualize the entire object. The valve morphology should determine the omniplane angle that is best suited to image it: the authors do not fit the valve to a predetermined omniplane angle.

A unique method for conceptualizing the aforementioned mitral valve anatomy is "the

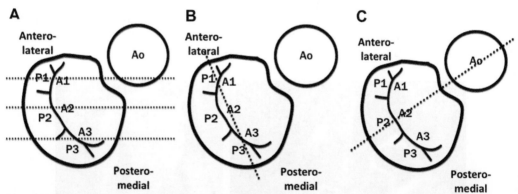

Fig. 2. (A) Viewing angles of the mitral valve. At 0°, advance or withdraw the probe in the mid-esophageal position to view each coaptation segment. (B) The bicommissural view at 60° to 90°. (C) The traditional grasping view for A2-P2 is at ~120°. The authors' protocol is as follows. Image at 0° from the most superior valve structure (lateral annulus) to the most inferior valve structure (medial annulus). Change omniplane to show bicommissural view (45°–70°). Once demonstrated, rotate the probe clockwise until the aortic valve is visualized: imaging plane will slice perpendicular to the commissural line along the anterior leaflet. Then rotate the probe counterclockwise until the posterior annulus is visualized, slicing perpendicular to the posterior leaflet. Next, change the omniplane to display the aorta and aortic valve in long axis (120°–140°): the A2-P2 scallops will be visualized. Rotate the probe counterclockwise to the left atrial appendage and then clockwise until the interatrial septum is visualized. Ao, aorta.

left-hand mitral rule." The left fist can be used to mimic the mitral valve anatomy, and may be helpful both in anticipation of imaging and in determining the optimal grasp view at the time of clip deployment (Fig. 3). This model serves as a simple imaging tool for understanding anatomy of the mitral valve and adjacent structures. With the hand in the shape of a fist, the dorsum of the fingers is the anterior leaflet and the visualized palm is the posterior leaflet. The thumb is the LAA, and the medial border of the hand is the interatrial septum. The right forearm then becomes the TEE probe and the flattened-out hand becomes the omniplane. With supination of the hand, the omniplane changes from 0° to 180°. Moving the right hand to the right is equivalent to clockwise rotation and moving it to the left is counterclockwise rotation. Anteroflexion is equivalent to moving the right hand superiorly and retroflexion, inferiorly. Lateral or medial wheel motion would move the forearm in an arc to the left or the right. This simple mitral and TEE model demonstrates how probe manipulation will or will not assist in visualization.

Beyond 2D TEE imaging, live 3D has become an essential part of mitral valve assessment. With the probe in mid-esophageal position at approximately 0° to 30°, the authors obtain 3D en-face reconstruction as a representation of the "surgeon's view" (Fig. 4). Live 3D TEE affords the added capability of visualizing the valve en face from either the left atrial or left ventricular aspect, which is particularly helpful in characterizing complex bileaflet disease. Several analyses of 3D TEE highlight the added sensitivity and accuracy in identification of mitral valve lesions, and data from the REALISM trial suggest lower MitraClip procedure time with the use of 3D TEE.[6–11]

With real-time 3D imaging, the need for transgastric views for procedural alignment has nearly been eliminated. Although baseline transgastric images are routinely acquired, they are not required in most cases. Rarely, if the chordal structures are interfering with a device in the left ventricle (LV), transgastric views may be helpful for visualizing the grasp or leaflet insertion.

In addition to mitral apparatus anatomy, the TEE provides assessment of MR severity and adjacent structures. Standard evaluation should also document flow reversal in the pulmonary vein, regurgitant volume, regurgitant fraction, proximal isovelocity surface area (PISA), and vena contracta. A comprehensive 2D TEE assessment before mitral valve intervention should also include visualization of the LAA to rule out thrombi, especially in patients with concomitant atrial fibrillation. The interatrial septum and left upper pulmonary vein should be well visualized in anticipation of the transseptal puncture.

As highlighted by the following discussion of procedural guidance, the echocardiographer serves a critical role in percutaneous mitral valve procedural success. The onus falls on the echocardiographer to develop a 3D understanding of the intracardiac anatomy, to allow for anticipatory guidance and optimal image acquisition in 2D planes and 3D volumes.

ECHOCARDIOGRAPHIC GUIDANCE OF THE MITRACLIP PROCEDURE

Live 2D TEE is critical to MitraClip procedural success. TEE offers complementary imaging with fluoroscopy guidance, including imaging of soft-tissue structures and real-time biplanar visualization to optimize each step of the procedural algorithm, from transseptal puncture to

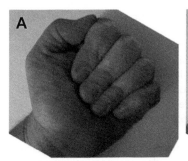 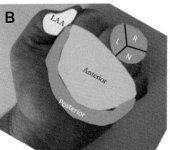 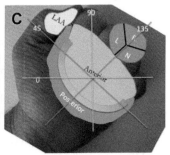

Fig. 3. Using the left hand as a teaching model for the mitral valve. (A) Palmar aspect of left hand modeling the atrial aspect of the mitral valve viewed from the left atrium. (B) Mitral valve structures over the closed left hand. (C) Omniplane displayed over the mitral model. The right hand (not shown) may also be used to mimic the TEE probe in this view. As the right hand supinates, the omniplane moves from 0° to 180°. Anterior, anterior mitral valve leaflet; L, left coronary cusp; LAA, left atrial appendage; N, noncoronary cusp; Posterior, posterior mitral valve leaflet; R, right coronary cusp.

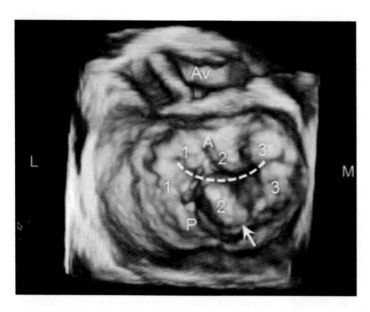

Fig. 4. Baseline TEE 3D en-face image of the mitral valve. The aortic valve (Av) is situated at the top of the image. The posterior leaflet (P) has 3 scallops starting laterally with 1 and moving medially to 3. The anterior leaflet (A) has the same numbering, defined by the adjacent posterior scallop. This patient has severe degenerative disease involving the P2 scallop with flail chordae.

navigation of the clip delivery system (CDS) and, ultimately, positioning of the clip with leaflet grasp. TEE also allows for assessment of residual MR and transvalvular gradient before clip release, thereby minimizing the risk of iatrogenic mitral stenosis and suboptimal reduction in regurgitation. Slipczuk and colleagues[12] have previously outlined a stepwise approach to TEE guidance of MitraClip insertion. The authors use a similar approach, but highlight here certain key differences in real-time guidance that are essential to optimizing outcomes in noncentral/eccentric disease.

Transseptal Puncture and Introduction of Delivery Sheath

As the traditional clinical trial target for Mitra-Clip deployment had been A2-P2, the main consideration for location of transseptal puncture had been the underlying type of MR: primary versus secondary. In general, the ideal puncture site is in the superior-posterior aspect of the interatrial septum. The goal is to be away from the aorta and at the appropriate height over the mitral annulus to manipulate the CDS in the left atrium. Subtle variations in the height of the puncture are made based on MR etiology.

Given that the line of coaptation for degenerative MR is typically above the mitral annulus, the recommended distance from CDS to annular plane is 4 to 4.5 cm, in contrast to functional MR, whereby the coaptation is often below the annulus and the recommended distance to the annulus is 3.5 to 4 cm. An additional layer of

complexity must be considered when approaching noncentral MR. Owing to the annulus angle being relative to the interatrial septum after transseptal puncture, and with introduction of the delivery sheath into the left atrium, the distance between the sheath tip and mitral annular plane increases as the sheath is advanced toward the lateral wall. As such, a standard transseptal puncture site may leave the CDS much further than 4.5 cm from the annular plane when approaching a lateral deployment target. The opposite is also true, whereby the CDS may be much closer than 3.5 cm from the annual plane if targeting a medial clip location. The conclusion is that the puncture site will need to be adjusted to accommodate variations from the standard A2-P2 location (**Fig. 5**).

The optimal views for localization of transseptal puncture are the short-axis aortic valve view (medial-lateral view) and the bicaval view (superior-inferior view). Moving actively between these views will aid in localization. Although current echocardiography systems allow biplane simultaneous imaging, the medial-lateral and superior-inferior views are not actually orthogonal; therefore, biplane should be used with caution (**Fig. 6**). Initially, after the operator has advanced the wire and transseptal sheath into the superior vena cava (SVC), TEE in the bicaval view will usually demonstrate saline contrast from the flush originating in the SVC. As the catheter is brought inferiorly, adjustments in omniplane and rotation of the probe should elongate the transseptal sheath to display the tip and, at least, initial shaft. Without displaying

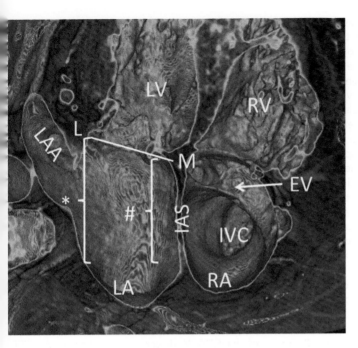

Fig. 5. Mitral valve annulus relative to interatrial septum. Implications for choosing transseptal point. Cardiac CT reconstruction. As the mitral valve annulus moves from medial (M) to lateral (L), the height from a given transseptal puncture will increase (*asterisk* vs *hash*). EV, Eustachian valve; IAS, interatrial septum; IVC, inferior vena cava; L, lateral; LA, left atrium; LAA, left atrial appendage; LV, left ventricle; M, medial; RA, right atrium; RV, right ventricle.

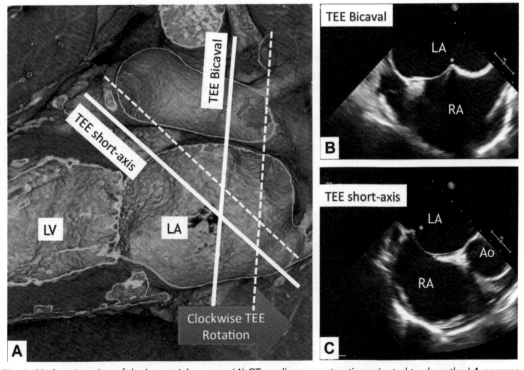

Fig. 6. X-plane imaging of the interatrial septum. (*A*) CT cardiac reconstruction oriented to show the LA perspective (also the TEE perspective) of the interatrial septum. (*B*) Bicaval view. (*C*) Short-axis view. Although the bicaval demonstrates superior and inferior orientation and the short axis the anterior and posterior orientation, the 2 views are not orthogonal. When the transseptal needle is moved posteriorly to gain height, the echocardiographer will lose the image in the short-axis view and will need to rotate the probe clockwise (moving from *solid white line* to *broken line*). *Asterisk*, tenting of the transseptal catheter before puncture.

the elongated view, the "tent" displayed may not actually be the distal end of the catheter, potentially resulting in an unintentional transseptal crossing point. Once the transseptal position is optimized and the septum is tented the TEE view is changed to a 4-chamber view to trace the anticipated course of the delivery sheath, and the annular distance is measured (see earlier discussion) (Fig. 7). The puncture site is then modified as appropriate for the clip target site.

Once the puncture site is identified, the puncture is performed with live TEE guidance in the short-axis view. A wire is guided into the left upper pulmonary vein. Continuous visualization is maintained, with simultaneous TEE and fluoroscopy, as the dilator and delivery sheath are advanced over the wire into the left atrium. Actively adjusting the rotation of the TEE probe to keep the entirety of the delivery sheath in view will reduce the risk of injury to the left atrial free wall. Once the dilator and sheath are safely and adequately positioned in the left atrium, the dilator is removed. The sheath generally extends approximately 2 cm across the interatrial septum. Depending on the size of the left atrium, the sheath will often need to be withdrawn slightly as the CDS is initially advanced into the left atrium (Fig. 8).

Insertion of the Clip Delivery System into the Left Atrium

The CDS is then advanced through the sheath into the left atrium under fluoroscopic guidance. The CDS is actively visualized exiting the sheath with TEE, again ensuring no damage to the left atrial posterior or lateral wall. The sheath may need to be retracted to allow the CDS adequate room in the left atrium to safely approach the mitral valve.

Tracking the trajectory of the CDS is an important imaging step in avoiding left atrial injury. This technique may be applied to guidance of any catheter through the left atrium. The omniplane is adjusted to elongate the CDS and at the same time display the lateral left atrial wall. In general, this is at an omniplane in the 40° to 70° range. While the CDS tip approaches the left pulmonary vein limbus, the TEE probe is rotated to display the orifice of the LAA and the CDS. The CDS may then be guided safely down to the mitral annulus with minimal risk of injury to the left atrial wall.

After the CDS is oriented toward the mitral valve, the omniplane is identified, which allows for visualization of the entire CDS in long axis. Typically this omniplane is most easily found by moving the structure of interest, the CDS, into the middle of the echocardiographic plane. One must keep in mind that the probe position in the esophagus is key; a very laterally oriented esophagus will only allow a foreshortened view of the CDS. With very vertical hearts, the TEE probe will need to be higher with retroflexion and rotation to achieve adequate visualization. This omniplane image foreshadows the TEE orientation for the grasp.

Clip Opening and Alignment Above the Mitral Valve

Once the CDS is positioned above the clip target, the clip is opened. The open clip is then oriented under echocardiographic guidance to be perpendicular to the line of coaptation at the anticipated clip site. Optimal orientation should result in clear visualization of the mitral valve leaflets and MitraClip gripper arms in the long-axis view (again, this view will

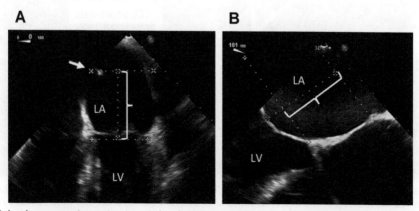

A   **B**

Fig. 7. Height above grasping point. In a 4-chamber view, usually at 0° (A) or occasionally in 150° to 170° range depending on probe location and heart rotation (B), measure the height from the transseptal needle tent to the anticipated grasp location. The patient viewed in A has degenerative disease, so the grasping point will be above the annulus, whereas in the patient with restricted leaflets (B), the grasping point will be below the annulus.

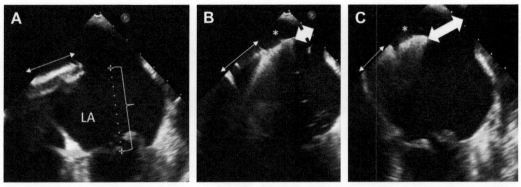

Fig. 8. TEE with 2D imaging of the steerable guide catheter (SGC) (*small double-sided arrow*) and clip delivery system (CDS) (*asterisk*) traversing the interatrial septum into the left atrium. (A) SGC advanced into the left atrium (LA) with height above mitral annulus measured (*bracket*). (B) The CDS is advanced into the LA through the SGC and approaches the LA wall (*double-sided arrow*). (C) The SGC is slightly withdrawn, creating a safe distance from the CDS to the atrial wall (*double-sided arrow*).

vary according to the clip target, but will generally be in a mid-esophageal probe position with beam angle in the 90°–140° range). The long-axis view is effective for anterior-posterior positioning of the clip, whereas the bicommissural view should be used for medial-lateral positioning (Fig. 9). En-face 3D imaging also facilitates positioning.

Initial positioning of the clip above the mitral valve is a technically challenging stage of echocardiographic MitraClip guidance. Noncentral disease and clip location adds another layer of complexity to this task. Live 3D TEE is particularly useful for this step of the procedure. An en-face view of the clip and CDS from the left atrial aspect allows for a more direct and effective method of determining the clip position. The clip position can also be assessed in biplane for simultaneous anterior-posterior and medial-lateral positioning (see Fig. 9). Although the surgical view with the aortic valve on top is a common method of displaying the 3D en-face view of the mitral valve, a more anatomic position may help to anticipate the grasp angle while approaching noncentral disease, whereby omniplane for medial is often more vertical (90°) and lateral is more horizontal (180°) (Fig. 10).

In determining the specific grasp point, it is essential to anticipate how the clip will change the overall configuration of the valve. Placing a clip on noncompliant leaflets may result in a higher than anticipated transvalvular gradient. Grasping redundant leaflet tissue may also bring an adjacent area closer and facilitate the subsequent grasp that would not be possible as an initial grasp. Anticipating the impact of an initial

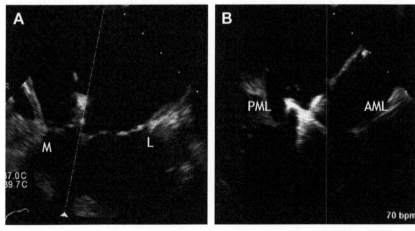

Fig. 9. Biplane imaging for alignment in the left atrium. (A) Bicommissural view with clip located medially. (B) Simultaneous long-axis view with clip oriented slightly posteriorly. AML, anterior mitral leaflet; L, lateral mitral annulus; M, medial mitral annulus; PML, posterior mitral leaflet.

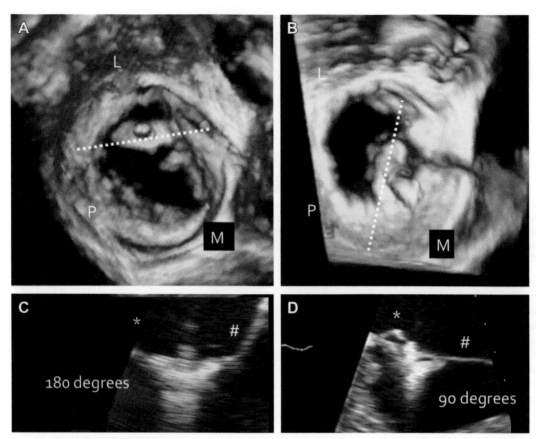

Fig. 10. TEE 3D en-face images rotated clockwise to a more anatomic representation of the actual orientation of the mitral valve in the body. (*A*) Patient with lateral degenerative disease. The clip is rotated almost horizontal in this view to orient the clip perpendicular to the line of coaptation. The corresponding grasp was performed at a horizontal omniplane of 180° (*C*). (*B*) Patient with very medial degenerative disease. The clip is rotated almost vertical to be perpendicular to the line of coaptation. The corresponding grasp was performed with a vertical omniplane of 90°. (Clip plane illustrated by *dashed line*) (*C*) Grasp view during lateral grasp in *A* with an omniplane of 180°. (*D*) Grasp view during medial grasp in *B* with an omniplane of 90°. *Hash,* anterior mitral valve leaflet; *asterisk,* posterior mitral valve leaflet; L, lateral; M, medial; P, posterior.

clip helps guide the strategy for both initial and subsequent clip deployment.

Advancement of the Clip into the Left Ventricle

After the clip alignment is optimized above the mitral valve, the clip is advanced through the valve into the LV under continuous TEE guidance to ensure appropriate trajectory, while avoiding chordal entanglement and monitoring for significant rotation (**Fig. 11**).

3D TEE is the primary means to confirm clip alignment once in the LV. Starting with an en-face view, by decreasing the gain the leaflets will fade as the more echogenic clip remains visualized. Minimal changes in orientation may then be made, or the clip may be withdrawn and repositioned if significantly distanced from the disease (**Fig. 12**). If 3D is suboptimal or not

available, transgastric short-axis views of the mitral valve will confirm orientation in the LV.

Grasping the Mitral Valve Leaflets

At this point, the clip is in the LV and is oriented perpendicular to the coaptation line at the location of the disease. No additional clip movement should be necessary before the grasp (**Fig. 13**). The echocardiographer now needs to find the view that displays the clip with arms extended, clip shaft, and leaflets. The authors recommend positioning the TEE probe to create an imaging plane whereby in a long-axis view the CDS, clip arms, and gripper arms are all in plane with the mitral leaflets (**Fig. 14**). This position will decrease the likelihood of the clip moving out of plane during the grasp.

Adequate time is necessary to ensure that the grasp view is optimal before and during the

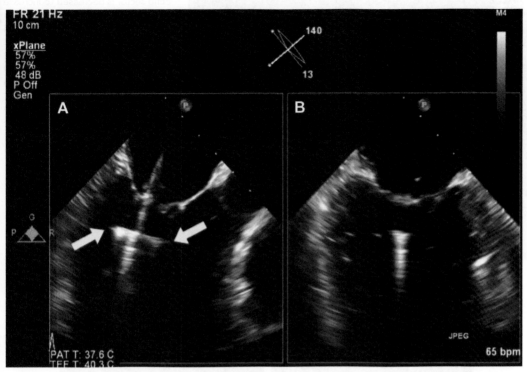

Fig. 11. Clip position using biplanar imaging after crossing into the LV. (A) Long axis for anterior-posterior positioning of the clip: gripper arms seen only in the long-axis view (*arrows*). (B) Bicommissural view for medial-lateral positioning (note gripper arms appropriately unseen).

grasp. Ideally the TEE image will display the CDS shaft and arms along with the leaflets. In the grasping view, measuring the leaflet lengths before grasp and after the initial grasp is performed, allowing confirmation of adequate grasp and seating of the leaflets (>4 mm of leaflet grasp is optimal, but >2 mm is essential to avoid clip detachment) (**Fig. 15**).[6,13] As the clip is brought up under the leaflets, the leaflets will float above the arms. Once the implanter is ready to grasp, a long image capture (up to 15 seconds) during the grasp allows the team to review the grasp before releasing the clip. Subtle movement of the leaflets that will compromise the grasp

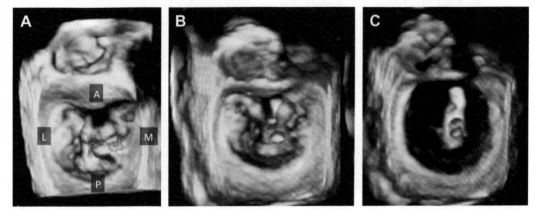

Fig. 12. Clip alignment in the LV. (A) Clip oriented in the left atrium, above A2-P2 scallops of a valve with severe posterior middle-scallop degenerative disease. (B) The clip has now been advanced into the LV and its arms are obscured by the leaflet tissue. (C) During the same image acquisition as in B, the gain is decreased and the more echodense clip is visible as the mitral leaflets essentially become transparent. As gain is varied, the orientation, perpendicular to the line of coaptation, may be confirmed.

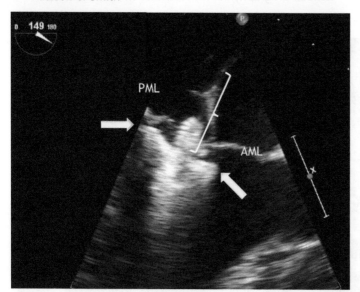

Fig. 13. Ideal imaging before grasp. Echo sector is decreased to increase temporal resolution. The clip arms (*arrows*), clip body, anterior and posterior mitral valve leaflets (AML and PML, respectively) and the shaft (*bracket*) are all visualized in one plane. As the clip is pulled up to the leaflets, the echocardiographer should anticipate a slight rotation of the TEE probe to maintain appropriate visualization of all structures.

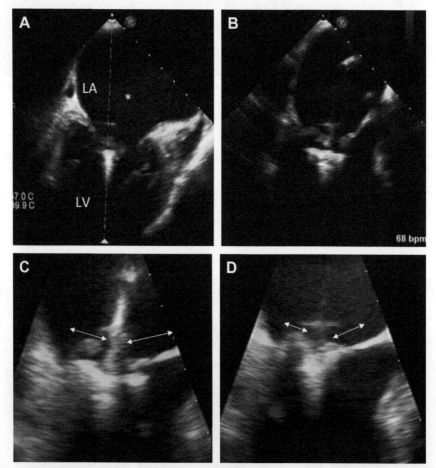

Fig. 14. Optimizing the grasp. (*A, B*) Biplane views, with *B* orthogonal to the vertical line in *A*. For optimization of the grasp it is ideal to have the shaft, leaflets, and clip arms in the same plane. The TEE position should be adjusted to create the closest image to *A*. Biplane will then confirm that a grasp view can be created just by moving the omniplane (*B*). (*C*) The image from *B* is zoomed and the leaflets are seen floating above the clip arms. With all of the key components in view, as the clip moves up it is very easy to maintain visualization. The leaflet lengths may be measured and compared with postgrasp (*D*). *, vertical line in *A*. *Arrows*, leaflet lengths before (*C*) and after (*D*) grasp.

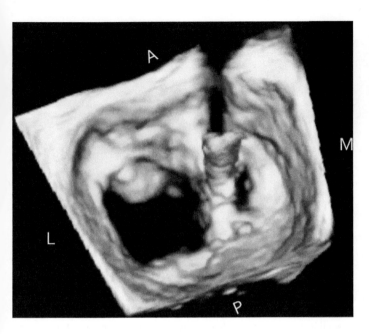

Fig. 15. En-face view of mitral valve following MitraClip grasp. A wide drape of the scallops is visualized over the clip arms. The wide drape over the clip is consistent with an appropriate amount of tissue within the grasp.

(such as a premature ventricular contraction) may be seen on this review.

A well-visualized grasp is the first step in ensuring a successful grasp. Following review of the grasp imaging, the authors rotate through the grasping view, 4-chamber view, and modified bicommissural view to confirm leaflet insertion. In addition to measurement of leaflet length, the leaflet should drape over the atrial aspect of the clip arm and mobility should be reduced. Live 3D en-face imaging can then be performed to visualize the resultant orifice (single vs double depending on eccentricity of clip placement), clip alignment, and insertion (Fig. 16). Following confirmation that anatomically there is sufficient leaflet insertion to safely release the clip, color flow Doppler will demonstrate whether adequate MR reduction has occurred. In the initial grasp assessment, the clip arms are not completely closed: this aids in visualizing the arms, leaflets, and grippers. As the color is turned on, the MR is visualized in the bicommissural view and the implanter tightens the clip arms. As the clip is tightened, coaptation increases and MR should further reduce. If esophageal views in 3D are not optimal, transgastric images at 0° to 30° for the short-axis view of the valve may be of additional value.

Spectral Doppler, 2D, and 3D volume color flow can be used to demonstrate reduction in regurgitation and consequent procedural success. Mitral regurgitation assessment is an integration of multiple variable observations. The modified mitral valve anatomy limits PISA as a quantitative measurement, although it will demonstrate the origin and trajectory of the MR. Color Doppler will demonstrate from where the residual leak is originating, and can help determine whether the clip needs to be moved or if a new clip will be necessary medially or laterally. If MR has been significantly reduced with intervention, pulmonary vein flow should no longer demonstrate reversal and a systolic predominant wave pattern is often seen. Color flow will be significantly reduced. A 3D vena contracta assessment may be the most objective assessment of orifice area; however, as temporal resolution decreases substantially, even on a small sector with 3D color, if the quality of the image is suboptimal then the 3D vena contracta should not be used.

The diastolic transmitral gradient should be measured through the residual orifice(s). The traditional cut-point for an acceptable post-MitraClip valvular stenosis is a mean transmitral gradient of at least 5 mm Hg. The authors recommend taking a patient-specific approach to the assessment of postintervention stenosis, with consideration of patients' functional status and resting heart rate. High-risk surgical patients with low functional status may tolerate resting mitral gradients in the 5- to 7-mm Hg range without symptoms. Patients with higher functional capacities may become symptomatic, as the gradient may increase with exercise. Valve area planimetry (particularly in the 3D en-face view) allows a direct measurement of valve area. Pressure half-time is not validated acutely

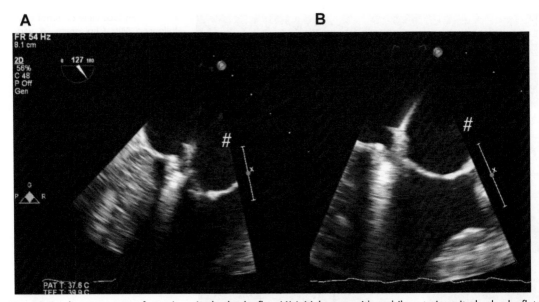

Fig. 16. Inadequate grasp of anterior mitral valve leaflet. (A) Initial grasp with mobile anterior mitral valve leaflet extending below the grasp arm. There is a very thin portion of the leaflet visualized at the anterior arm. The clip was released and regrasped. (B) Second grasp with now adequate grasp of the anterior leaflet. There is much less mobility of the anterior leaflet with the thicker portion of the leaflet grasped. #, anterior mitral leaflet.

and, given its dependence on left atrial compliance, the authors do not use it for acute valve area assessment.

If the initial result is suboptimal from the standpoint of regurgitation, the appearance of the residual regurgitant jet will determine how to proceed with intervention.[12] If the MR reduction after first grasp is not sufficient there are several potential options that can be used to modify the procedure, including: (1) continue with clip deployment in the current position and plan for additional adjacent clip(s); or (2) move the initial clip position and reassess for need of additional clip(s). The echocardiographer must anticipate how each planned clip will affect the leaflet morphology around the clip. Each clip placement will affect the ability and success of the subsequent clip placement.

Releasing the Clip and Additional Assessment
Once the clip position and leaflet seating are confirmed, and color flow Doppler interrogation is complete, the clip is released. Additional clips will then be placed with echocardiographic

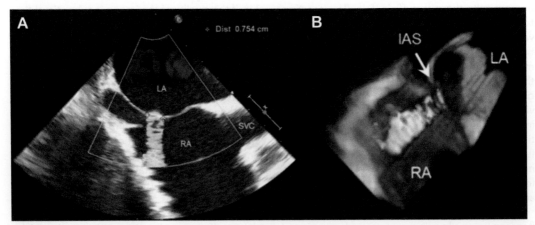

Fig. 17. (A, B) Evaluating the diameter of an iatrogenic atrial septal defect (iASD) after removal of the clip delivery system. This patient has a left-to-right shunt through the iASD. (A) Bicaval view of the interatrial septum, 2D with color Doppler. (B) 3D with color Doppler of interatrial septum. IAS, interatrial septum; LA, left atrium; RA, right atrium.

guidance as outlined earlier. After the MitraClip procedure is completed, the CDS is removed. Repeat 2D/3D and color flow Doppler should be performed with the clip(s) implanted. Specific attention needs to be given to the shaft of the CDS as it is removed from the left atrium. The tip of the CDS needs to be guided out of the left atrium, essentially in a reversal of how it was placed, to avoid left atrial injury.

A postprocedure iatrogenic atrial septal defect (iASD) may be evaluated with color flow Doppler (Fig. 17). As the authors have previously reported,[14] the incidence of persistent iASDs following MitraClip is similar to that of other transseptal interventional procedures (27%). Only in rare cases such as large residual iASD, or significant right-to-left shunting with oxygen desaturation, is closure clearly indicated. More recently, Schueler and colleagues[15] have identified persistence of iASD at 50% when TEE is used. The utility of closing small iASDs remains unclear.

SUMMARY

As percutaneous intervention for mitral valve regurgitation continues to expand, the importance and reliance on imaging guidance will grow in parallel. MitraClip is the clearest contemporary example of this coevolution, with significant experience garnered from the interventional community now that the device has wide commercial availability. Many of the best-practice approaches outlined in this article may be successfully applied to the myriad options for percutaneous mitral valve intervention currently in the development pipeline. TEE training must emphasize a "full-volume" understanding of the mitral valve to allow imagers to comfortably and seamlessly guide procedures. Effective imaging support optimizes intervention planning, safety, and procedural success.

REFERENCES

1. Nishimura RA, Otto CM, Bonow RO, et al. 2014 AHA/ACC guideline for the management of patients with valvular heart disease: a report of the American College of Cardiology/American Heart Association Task Force on Practice Guidelines. J Am Coll Cardiol 2014; 63:e57–185.

2. Franzen O, Baldus S, Rudolph V, et al. Acute outcomes of MitraClip therapy for mitral regurgitation in high-surgical-risk patients: emphasis on adverse valve morphology and severe left ventricular dysfunction. Eur Heart J 2010;31:1373–81.

3. Feldman T, Foster E, Glower DD, et al. Percutaneous repair or surgery for mitral regurgitation. N Engl J Med 2011;364:1395–406.

4. Singh GD, Smith TW, Rogers JH. Multi-MitraClip therapy for severe degenerative mitral regurgitation: "anchor" technique for extremely flail segments. Catheter Cardiovasc Interv 2015;86(2):339–46.

5. Foster GP, Isselbacher EM, Rose GA, et al. Accurate localization of mitral regurgitant defects using multiplane transesophageal echocardiography. Ann Thorac Surg 1998;65:1025–31.

6. Grewal J, Mankad S, Freeman WK, et al. Real-time three-dimensional transesophageal echocardiography in the intraoperative assessment of mitral valve disease. J Am Soc Echocardiogr 2009;22:34–41.

7. Wei J, Hsiung MC, Tsai SK, et al. The routine use of live three-dimensional transesophageal echocardiography in mitral valve surgery: clinical experience. Eur J Echocardiogr 2010;11:14–8.

8. La Canna G, Arendar I, Maisano F, et al. Real-time three-dimensional transesophageal echocardiography for assessment of mitral valve functional anatomy in patients with prolapse-related regurgitation. Am J Cardiol 2011;107:1365–74.

9. Thompson KA, Shiota T, Tolstrup K, et al. Utility of three-dimensional transesophageal echocardiography in the diagnosis of valvular perforations. Am J Cardiol 2011;107:100–2.

10. Ben Zekry S, Nagueh SF, Little SH, et al. Comparative accuracy of two- and three-dimensional transthoracic and transesophageal echocardiography in identifying mitral valve pathology in patients undergoing mitral valve repair: initial observations. J Am Soc Echocardiogr 2011;24:1079–85.

11. Biner S, Perk G, Kar S, et al. Utility of combined two-dimensional and three-dimensional transesophageal imaging for catheter-based mitral valve clip repair of mitral regurgitation. J Am Soc Echocardiogr 2011;24:611–7.

12. Slipczuk L, Siegel RJ, Jilaihawi H, et al. Optimizing procedural outcomes in percutaneous mitral valve therapy using transesophageal imaging: a stepwise analysis. Expert Rev Cardiovasc Ther 2012;10:901–16.

13. Guarracino F, Baldassarri R, Ferro B, et al. Transesophageal echocardiography during MitraClip(R) procedure. Anesth Analg 2014;118:1188–96.

14. Smith T, McGinty P, Bommer W, et al. Prevalence and echocardiographic features of iatrogenic atrial septal defect after catheter-based mitral valve repair with the MitraClip system. Catheter Cardiovasc Interv 2012;80:678–85.

15. Schueler R, Ozturk C, Wedekind JA, et al. Persistence of iatrogenic atrial septal defect after interventional mitral valve repair with the MitraClip system: a note of caution. JACC Cardiovasc Interv 2015;8:450–9.

Use of Computed Tomography to Guide Mitral Interventions

Vladimir Jelnin, MD[a],*, Chad Kliger, MD[b],
Fabio Zucchetta, MD[c], Carlos E. Ruiz, MD, PhD[a]

KEYWORDS

- CTA • Fluoroscopy • 3D reconstruction • Virtual planning • Fusion

---

KEY POINTS

- Improved CTA temporal and spatial resolution have afforded the opportunity to evaluate cardiac structure and function and, now integral in characterizing MV disease.
- 3D cardiac reconstruction allows for anatomic evaluation of the MV apparatus including prosthetics devices and important surrounding structures.
- Fusion imaging allows for the merger of pre-procedural CTA with live fluoroscopy.
- Virtual procedural planning using fusion imaging enables the selection of best access approach(es) and device(s).
- Landmarks can be overlaid directly onto fluoroscopy for procedural guidance, particularly helpful during MV interventions where there is a lack of fluoroscopic mitral landmarks.

INTRODUCTION

Cardiac computed tomographic angiography (CTA) has focused traditionally on the evaluation of coronary artery disease. Overall, CTA has been underused owing to a multitude of reasons: the need for advanced equipment not universally available, the requirement for contrast media and ionizing radiation, the presence of limited reimbursement, and more important, the expertise required for the acquisition and postprocessing/reconstruction. It is not considered the gold standard imaging modality for the assessment of the mitral valve (MV) apparatus by most interventionalists and imaging specialists. However, its ability to provide high spatial resolution images compared with alternative modalities offers the unique potential for anatomic evaluation of the MV. With increasing use of CTA for structural heart disease and the widespread adoption of fusion imaging technology allowing the merger of preprocedural CTA with fluoroscopy, our ability to plan and guide complex MV interventions is now possible. This article details the role of CTA in imaging of MV disease and support for transcatheter therapies.

IMAGING FOR MITRAL VALVE INTERVENTIONS

Echocardiography, both transthoracic and transesophageal (TEE), is the gold standard imaging modality for the assessment of MV disease and guidance for intervention, whether surgical or transcatheter. TEE is the most widely accepted modality of choice.[1–4] It provides essential functional information while displaying blood flow (ie, color Doppler); advances in 3-dimensional

---

[a] Division of Structural and Congenital Heart Disease, Heart and Vascular Hospital, Hackensack University Medical Center, 30 Prospect Avenue, Hackensack, NJ 07601, USA; [b] Department of Cardiothoracic Surgery, Division of Structural and Congenital Heart Disease, Hofstra University School of Medicine, Lenox Hill Hospital, North Shore LIJ Health System, 130 East 77th Street, 4th Floor Black Hall, New York, NY 10075, USA; [c] Department of Cardiology, Thoracic and Vascular Sciences, Division of Cardiac Surgery, University of Padua, Via Giustiniani 2, Padua 35128, Italy
* Corresponding author. 188 E 78th Street, 8B, New York, NY 10075.
E-mail address: vjelnin@gmail.com

Intervent Cardiol Clin 5 (2016) 33–43
http://dx.doi.org/10.1016/j.iccl.2015.08.003
2211-7458/16/$ – see front matter © 2016 Elsevier Inc. All rights reserved.

(3D) TEE offer enhanced visualization cardiac of abnormalities, as well as interventional equipment in real time. Additionally, intraprocedural complications such as perforations, tamponade, and device embolization can be assessed without delay.

Interest in CTA for assessment and procedural guidance of MV disease has grown significantly with the evolution of this technology. With the advent of electron beam CTA, its major utility was quantification of calcification for coronary disease evaluation.[5,6] In 2000, the introduction of multidetector CTA further established its role in the assessment of coronary disease.[7,8] Subsequent improvements in temporal and spatial resolution have afforded the opportunity for CTA to evaluate cardiac structure and function and, more recently integral to characterize both native and prosthetic cardiac valves; in particular for the MV,[9–14] this includes the presence of mitral annular calcification, leaflet thickening and calcification, leaflet prolapse, and rupture and/or thickening of the chordae tendinae and papillary muscles. Although challenges remain, such as limited visualization of the MV owing to the relatively minor thickness of the leaflets and chordae tendinae, high-velocity cardiac motion, and significant artifacts from the surrounding calcification, the usefulness of the technology continues to mature.[15–18]

Currently, the predominant literature on CTA for guidance of structural heart interventions is dedicated to TAVR.[19–23] Three-dimensional volume rendering (VR) of the vasculature can assess for tortuosity, and measurements can accurately be performed to determine atherosclerotic disease and its ability to accommodate delivery sheath, as well as alternative access routes. Measurements of the valve complex are important to minimize complications particularly paravalvular regurgitation and coronary occlusion, with CTA providing more accurate measurements than 2-dimensional (2D) transthoracic echocardiography or TEE. Furthermore, manipulation of images can identify the optimal fluoroscopic views for transcatheter valve implantation. More recently, the use of CTA for MV has expanded to the treatment of paravalvular leaks (PVL)[24–28] and prosthetic valve dysfunction with valve-in-valve implantation. The most common MV intervention, the Mitraclip (Abbott, Abbott Park IL), continues to rely on the TEE for procedural planning and guidance.

The usefulness of CTA for the guidance of MV interventions can be divided into 3 categories:

- Image acquisition and diagnostics;
- Preprocedural planning; and
- Intraprocedural guidance.

Image Acquisition and Diagnostics

The importance of quality source CT data should not be underestimated; the reliability of measurements and quality of image reconstruction is proportionally dependent on the cross-sectional images. Factors affecting data quality include body habitus, increased and/or irregular heart rate (arrhythmia), and artifacts from extensive calcification and/or prosthetic devices such as postoperative metal clips or prostheses. Sufficient contrast enhancement in the area of interest, that is, the left atrium and ventricle in the case of MV assessment, during acquisition is essential.

Image acquisition starts with evaluation of the patient's personal data. Body size with an increased body mass index is usually the major component of a suboptimal study. Adjustments of the x-ray tube power setting (mA, KV) according to the scanner manufacturer's protocols can improve image quality. Heart rate is another equally important parameter. Coronary CTA acquisition protocols require a heart rate of approximately 60 bpm or less to reduce motion artifacts; structural CTA follows the same rules. Administration of β-blockers (oral or intravenous) is useful to decrease motion artifacts. The use of helical acquisition with retrospective electrocardiographic (ECG) gating allows for the reconstruction of multiple phases of the cardiac cycle in the search for the best possible, motion artifact–free image. Furthermore, adequate contrast enhancement depends on optimal transit time for the contrast to reach the left heart from the antecubital vein. This time can be calculated easily using the same protocol for the coronary CTA. The most common intravenous site is antecubital with an 18-G catheter and a contrast volume of 75 to 90 mL (1 mL/Kg) injected at the rate of 5 to 6 mL/s. A saline chaser is not required unless concomitant coronary evaluation is needed.

There are 2 main acquisition protocols, namely, retrospective ECG gating with multiple phase reconstruction and prospective ECG gating with acquisition during a preselected single phase of the cardiac cycle. Prospective ECG gating has a significantly lesser radiation dose compared with the helical acquisition (2–3 vs 12–15 mSv) and is typically used in younger patients and when repeat surveillance scans are likely to be required. Single phase acquisition for the MV, however, provides limited information; it is usually acquired in end-diastole and shows the MV leaflets during opening, with no information during valve systole. Helical acquisition allows reconstruction during the entire cardiac cycle. Reconstruction sets have from 10 to 20 phases equally spaced between the R–R interval of the ECG. This data after VR, if displayed in the cine mode, can provide 4-dimensional images of the MV in motion during the entire cardiac cycle, demonstrating the location of valvular defect with a high level of precision. CT has significantly higher spatial resolution than echocardiography[29] and the proper use of VR with accurate contrast subtraction allows improved visualization of the mitral apparatus.

Preprocedural Planning

Three-dimensional anatomic evaluation of the MV apparatus, including prosthetic devices and surrounding structures, is critical. Common classification of location and components are typically visualized from the surgeon's view where the valve is seen from the left atrium with the aortic valve placed cephalad. Using a clock-face approach, 12 o'clock represents the mitral–aortic fibrous continuity and from there, the remaining components: 3 o'clock corresponds with the area of the interatrial septum, 6 o'clock with the posterolateral free wall, and 9 o'clock with the left atrial appendage (Fig. 1). The remaining components of the MV can be identified in addition to its relationships with

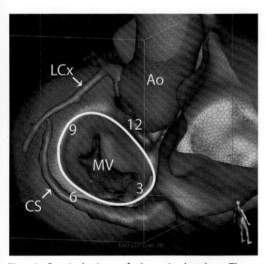

Fig. 1. Surgical view of the mitral valve. Three-dimensional volume-rendered cardiac reconstruction showing the mitral and aortic complexes from a posterior view. The mitral-aortic fibrous continuity is located at 12 o'clock with the interatrial septum at 3 o'clock, posterolateral free wall at 6 o'clock, and left atrial appendage at 9 o'clock. Ao, aorta; CS, coronary sinus; LCx, left circumflex coronary artery; MV, mitral valve.

the left circumflex artery, coronary sinus, and left ventricular (LV) outflow tract.

Evaluation of prosthetic valves and detection of pannus, prosthetic leaflet thickening, thrombus adherence and/or calcification, abnormal leaflet mobility, and the presence of surrounding pseudoaneurysm or PVL(s) can be performed. For PVLs around surgical prostheses, CTA can be used to determine its size and shape, course with many having serpiginous tracts, degree of surrounding calcification, interaction with other cardiac structures, and overall best access strategies for transcatheter repair. For mitral PVLs located along the intraatrial septum, it is sometimes difficult to access via an antegrade transseptal approach owing to the required catheter angulation, with the most favorable crossing path being via a retrograde transapical or transaortic approach.

The latest advances in the CTA post processing and more recently CTA–fluoroscopy fusion imaging have allowed for virtual planning. A 3D model of the heart can be generated with the MV anatomy and pathology of interest identified, along with extracardiac structures. Using this model, the interventionalist can select the most direct and potentially safest access approach and predict the type and size of device required. Using CTA–fluoroscopy fusion software (HeartNavigator, Philips Healthcare, Best, The Netherlands), a 3D model can be generated by automatic segmentation of the CTA data with each structure color coded (Fig. 2).

Manual correction and/or addition of structures can be performed when adjustment is needed. The operator also has the option to adjust the contour and even build the entire structure de novo. Background and surrounding tissues can be removed entirely or remain visible as maximal intensity projection rendering with variable density. The cardiac model can also be displayed either partially, structure by structure, or in its entirety, depending on the preference for analysis. Tools that allow for free manual rotation, application of cut planes, zoom options, and measurements provide for comprehensive review.

The MV apparatus, despite its many described challenges to visualize, can still be analyzed using this cardiac CTA postprocessing technique. The 3D reconstruction allows for clear positioning of oblique planes through the MV with good visualization and the ability to measure appropriate MV anatomy. Measurements can be performed of the MV leaflets (Fig. 3) and the "posterior shelf" (Fig. 4), the space lateral to the posterior mitral leaflet and

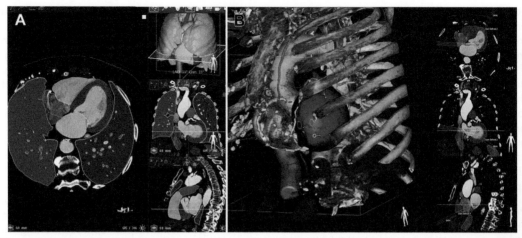

Fig. 2. Three-dimensional (3D) cardiac model for procedural planning. (A) Segmentation of cardiac and thoracic anatomy is performed automatically with different coded colors on the standard axial computed tomography view (main window). Right panel contains the views (from the top) of 3D reconstructed model, coronal, and sagittal views, respectively. Manual correction and/or addition of structures can be performed if required. (B) Main window (left) demonstrates 3D model of the heart and it positioning inside the chest. Ribs, sternum, and the spine are rendered using maximum intensity projection technique. (Right) Axial, coronal, and sagittal views, respectively (from the top).

LV myocardium deemed the potential landing zone for transcatheter MV technologies. Identification of this area using simple 2D plans is problematic and does not adequately illustrate the anatomy through its entire length. In contrast, 3D visualization allows complete MV apparatus inspection and measurements, and can aid in

prediction of prosthesis compatibility with real anatomy.

Visualization and assessment of 3D interrelations of the papillary muscles and chordae tendineae is another challenge. Chordae usually can be seen in limited numbers owing to their size and the limited CTA spatial resolution. Even a

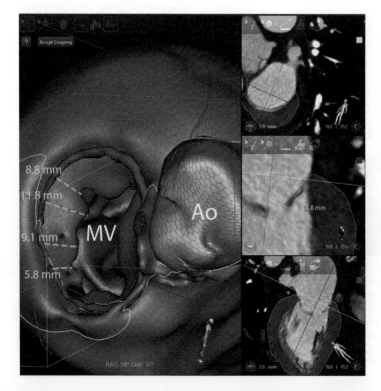

Fig. 3. Complex 3-dimensional (3D) shape of the mitral valve (MV) leaflets. All the measurement (in green) are performed on oblique planes (right panel) positioning using 3D visualization of the entire leaflet placed perpendicular to the annulus. Measurement lines are not parallel to each other, but rather perpendicular to the mitral annulus (Red shape). Ao, aorta.

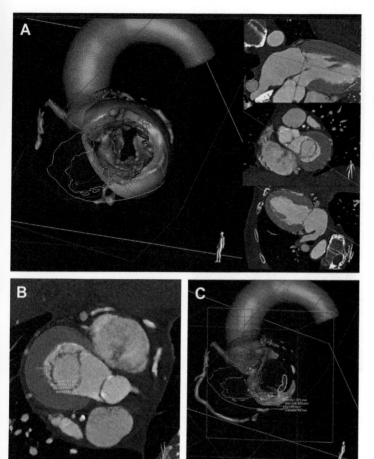

Fig. 4. Three-dimensional (3D) identification of the "posterior shelf" for transcatheter mitral valve implantation. (*A*) 3D positioning of the mitral annular plane lateral to the P2 with the reference 3 oblique planes (*right panel*). (*B*) Multiple measurements performed on the annular plane. (*C*) Visualization of the "posterior shelf" on 3D imaging.

good quality CTA is capable of showing only a small number compared with the real anatomic specimen. Papillary muscles are usually well seen, but assessment using 2D imaging shows only the structures captured in the 2D plane; constant manipulations with the oblique plane are needed to see all the muscles and to fully evaluate 3D interrelations. With 3D review, however, these manipulations are not necessary (Fig. 5).

Once a detailed anatomic review is performed, planning continues with the selection of access approach. The MV can be accessed from 3 different directions: antegrade transseptal, retrograde transaortic, and retrograde transapical through LV puncture, either operative or percutaneous. The feasibility of the each approach depends on the anatomic defect location, condition of the surrounding structures, and operator preference and experience (Fig. 6).

Next after segmentation, landmarks can be placed on important cardiac and extracardiac structures. Markers can be positioned in 3D, providing precise location during manipulation, and subsequently overlaid onto fluoroscopy during the interventional procedure for guidance. A path can be displayed connecting landmarks to provide a visual track for needle, wire, and/or device direction between 2 points in 3D (Fig. 7A). Planning for access, such as site-specific transseptal or transapical, can be performed using this technique.

Virtual placement of devices can also be accomplished within structural heart defects with varying sizes to aid in device determination (Fig. 7B and C). This option may be helpful for choosing the most appropriate placement of the prosthetic valves for the patient's anatomy, that is, transcatheter valve-in-valve, valve-in-ring, and newer transcatheter mitral valve replacement technologies. Models of the prosthesis built to scale and shape will help to evaluate the interactions with the patient's anatomy before the procedure (Fig. 8).

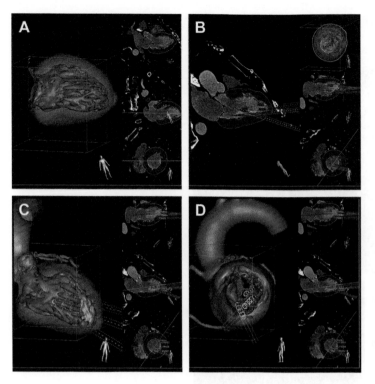

Fig. 5. Three-dimensional (3D) visualization of remainder of mitral valve apparatus. (A) 3D reconstruction of the papillary muscles. (B) Multiple oblique planes show the limited view of the papillary muscles. (C) Major papillary muscles are marked with different color marker "cylinders" following their 3D position within the left ventricle in lateral view. (D) Review of the same marked papillary muscles in the apical view (short axis).

Intraprocedural Guidance: Computed Tomographic Angiography–Fluoroscopy Fusion Imaging

Fluoroscopy remains as the foundation for imaging guidance. It, however, provides poor characterization of nonradiopaque structures and has the ability to provide only 2D projections. With fusion imaging, the segmented images with landmarks from the CTA, as detailed, can be registered and directly overlaid onto fluoroscopy. Improved spatial information from CTA provides more precise localization of abnormalities through incorporation of 3D data while preserving the temporal resolution of fluoroscopy. Real-time imaging guidance within the cardiac catheterization laboratory has the potential to provide improved accuracy and safety, while reducing radiation exposure, contrast volume, and procedural time.

The 2 modalities are registered with one another by matching the 3D position and scale of both images. Registration can be performed using contrast injection within the aorta or coronary arteries during angiography and then matching the location with the same

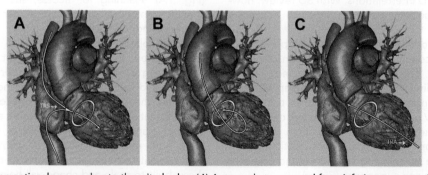

Fig. 6. Interventional approaches to the mitral valve. (A) Antegrade transseptal from inferior vena cava (most common) or superior vena cava. (B) Retrograde transaortic from the aorta crossing the aortic valve. (C) Retrograde transapical through left ventricular puncture.

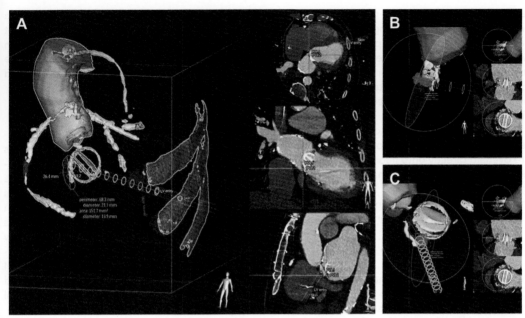

Fig. 7. Transapical puncture planning using landmarking tool and virtual device implantation. (A) Three-dimensional (3D) reconstruction with landmarks placed at skin entry, left ventricular entry, and structural heart defect (paravalvular leak [PVL]) around a mechanical mitral valve. A blue cylinder is generated to help direct needle entry through the chest wall into the left ventricle. (B, C) Virtual device implantation of an Amplatzer Vascular Plug II (St Jude Medical, Minneapolis, MN) within a mitral PVL.

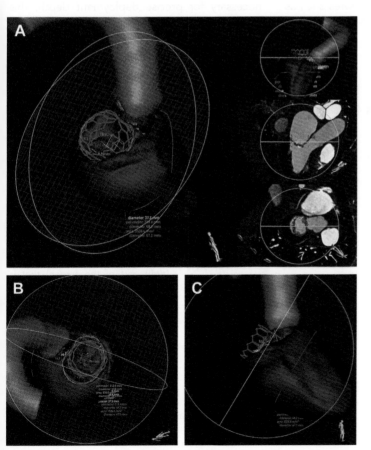

Fig. 8. Virtual planning for transcatheter mitral valve interventions. (A) Model of the mitral prosthesis (red stent lattice) positioned in the native mitral annulus (blue ring), main window, 3-dimensional reconstruction; right panel, visualization in oblique planes (middle and bottom windows). (B, C) Review of the virtual prosthesis from different angles. Yellow circle is the plane of the mitral annulus and the green circle represents a perpendicular plane. (C) In this view, the mitral annular plane shown as the straight line, representing the best C-arm position for the valve deployment. The appropriate depth of prosthesis implantation can be determined.

reconstructed structure on CTA image or by noncontrast registration using internal markers, namely, easily identifiable prosthetic material within the heart, such as the metal frame of a surgical prosthetic valves or pacemaker wires (Fig. 9). In some cases, extensive calcification of the aorta, coronary arteries, or the valve annulus can be used.

Once merged to fluoroscopy, outline of the reconstructed CTA image along with landmarks are overlaid directly onto fluoroscopy. With rotation of the C-arm, the CTA image and landmarks move in real time, providing 3D anatomic information during the procedure. Fusion imaging can facilitate access and interventional procedure.

Access

Site-specific transseptal puncture can be performed by placement of a landmark on the interatrial septum, with a predetermined height above the MV, often required for MV interventions (Fig. 10). In addition, guidance for percutaneous transapical access can be performed with placement of landmarks on the site of skin entry, LV entry, and MV defect (Fig. 11). Needle positioning away from important structures such as the ribs, coronary arteries, and lungs are essential to reduce complications.

The ability to create the safe and visible corridor—"cylinder"—for needle entry cannot be underemphasized. The same landmarks can also be used for transapical closure as the Amplatzer device (St Jude Medical) is positioned within the access tract (Fig. 12).

Intervention

The usefulness of fusion guidance can be appreciated fully by such procedures as percutaneous PVL closure and mitral valve-in-valve implantation, especially when fluoroscopic markers are not present (Figs. 13 and 14). CTA provides exclusively anatomic information with a high level of accuracy; however, it is unable to assess the success of leak closure owing to lack of flow dynamic information. Implantation of transcatheter heart valves within existing failed surgical mitral prostheses is being increasing performed on patient high risk for reoperative surgical replacement.

Procedural success depends on appropriate sizing of the prosthesis and identifying the valve/landing zone for implantation. CTA imaging is able to predict the best possible C-arm position perpendicular to the mitral annular plane necessary for precise deployment depth; this positioning is key in patients with radiolucent mitral prostheses.

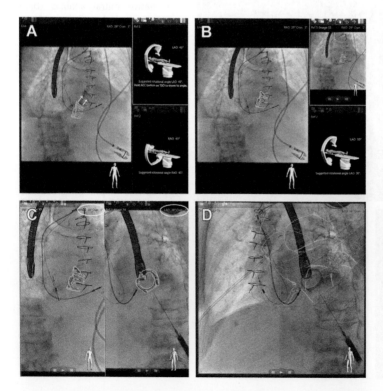

Fig. 9. Registration of computed tomography data with live fluoroscopy using internal markers (mitral valve prosthesis). (A) In the right anterior oblique C-arm projection, the rendered prosthetic valve frame is moved manually to match the frame on the fluoroscopy image (white arrows). (B) Position of matching valve frame on both imaging modalities is accepted for this C-arm position. (C) Position of the C-arm is changed to the left anterior oblique projection (right part of the screen) that is greater than 30° from the first projection and the valve frame is moved again to match the image on fluoroscopy. (D) After correlating in both C-arm views, registration is accepted and entire 3-dimensional reconstructed cardiac model is overlaid directly onto fluoroscopy with computed tomographic angiography image following the C-arm position.

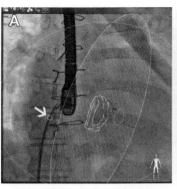
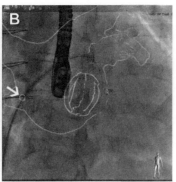

Fig. 10. Guidance of transseptal puncture. (A) Marker (blue circle, white arrow) is placed at the precise location on 3-dimensional reconstructed computed tomographic angiography overlaid onto the live fluoroscopy to aid in transseptal puncture. The target is a paravalvular leak identified next to the prosthetic mitral valve (MV; red dot). (B) The catheter with guidewire is visualized within the left atrium across the intended site of access. Contours of the left atrium and mechanical MV (yellow outline) can be seen easily on the fluoroscopy image.

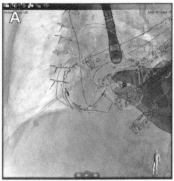
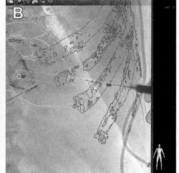

Fig. 11. Guidance of percutaneous transapical puncture. (A) Left anterior oblique C-arm projection with transapical access cylinder (blue circles) visualized en face with superimposed landmarks of skin entry, left ventricular entry, and center of mitral valve prosthesis. The entire needle path is seen as the "bullseye" allowing the precise needle positioning for puncture. (B) Anteroposterior C-arm projection to confirm needle trajectory within the predetermined access cylinder (blue circles).

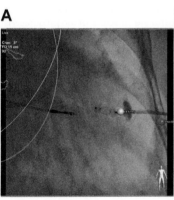
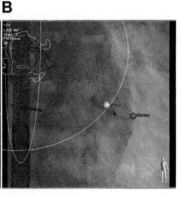

Fig. 12. Guidance for percutaneous transapical access closure. (A) Positioning of an Amplatzer Vascular Plug II (St Jude Medical) can be visualized with the distal disk placed on the endocardial surface and the proximal disk on the epicardial surface. The left ventricular entry landmark (orange dot) identifies the epicardial surface. Red marker is at the site of skin puncture. (B) The device has been fully deployed.

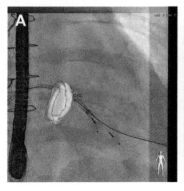
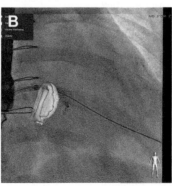

Fig. 13. Fusion guidance for paravalvular leak (PVL) closure. (A) Arteriovenous (AV) rail from transseptal and transapical access is created and antegrade delivery sheath crossed the PVL (red marker) into the left ventricle with 2 closure devices (AVP II). (B) Delivery sheath is withdrawn back to the left atrium with both closure devices positioned within the PVL defect. The safety wire (AV rail) remains across the leak. The mechanical mitral valve is identified in yellow.

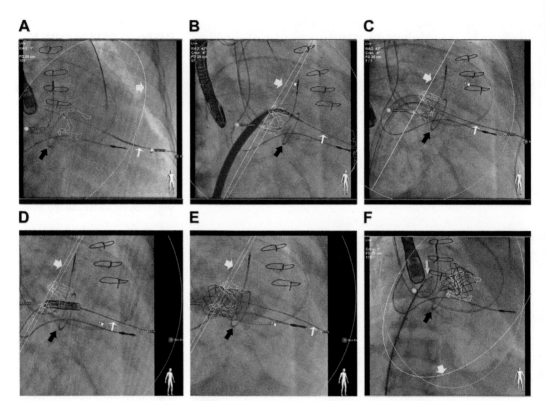

Fig. 14. Fusion guidance for valve-in-valve implantation within a radiolucent mitral prosthesis. (A) Transseptal and transapical access to the left heart were performed and an arteriovenous (AV) rail created. Blue dot, transseptal puncture; white arrow, transapical catheter; red marker, skin entry; yellow marker, LV entry. The yellow arrow is pointing to the mitral annular plane (*yellow ellipse*), the black arrow is pointing to the tricuspid incomplete valvular ring, not to be confused with the mitral valve (MV); the MV frame is radiolucent and the structure of the prosthesis is seen exclusively on computed tomographic angiography overlay (*white contour*). (B) Sheath/dilator introduced to the MV via transseptal approach over the AV rail. (C) Valve delivery sheath is introduced into mitral prosthesis. (D) Prosthetic valve (Melody, Medtronic Inc) is delivered to the deployment position defined by the annular plane (*yellow arrow*) and failed prosthetic valve frame (*white contour*). (E) Balloon inflation during valve deployment. (F) Final result. The deployed prosthesis is in a good position inside the failed surgical valve. Transseptal puncture site (*blue marker*) is closed with an Amplatzer Septal Occluder (St Jude Medical) device (*blue arrow*).

SUMMARY

The ability of cardiac CTA to guide structural heart interventions has evolved significantly through the years, and more recently in the MV space. In conjunction with CTA–fluoroscopy fusion imaging technology, it has opened new possibilities in MV procedures with improved preprocedural planning and intraprocedural guidance. Given the lack of fluoroscopic landmarks of the mitral apparatus and the continued growth of native MV device technologies, the value of CTA will continue to develop.

REFERENCES

1. Nishimura RA, Otto CM, Bonow RO, et al. 2014 AHA/ACC guideline for the management of patients with valvular heart disease: executive summary: a report of the American college of cardiology/American heart association task force on practice guidelines. J Am Coll Cardiol 2014; 63(22):2438–88.

2. Hahn RT, Abraham T, Adams MS, et al. Guidelines for performing a comprehensive transesophageal echocardiographic examination: recommendations from the American Society of Echocardiography and the Society of Cardiovascular Anesthesiologists. J Am Soc Echocardiogr 2013; 26(9):921–64.

3. Naqvi TZ. Echocardiography in percutaneous valve therapy. JACC Cardiovasc Imaging 2009;2(10): 1226–37.

4. Cavalcante JL, Rodriguez LL, Kapadia S, et al. Role of echocardiography in percutaneous mitral valve interventions. JACC Cardiovasc Imaging 2012;5(7): 733–46.

5. Detrano R. Coronary artery scanning using electron beam computed tomography. Am J Card Imaging 1996;10(2):97–100.

6. Becker C, Knez A, Ohnesorge B, et al. Visualization and quantification of coronary calcifications with electron beam and spiral computed tomography. Eur Radiol 2000;10(4):629–35.

7. Nasir K, Budoff MJ, Post WS, et al. Electron beam CT versus helical CT scans for assessing coronary calcification: current utility and future directions. Am Heart J 2003;146(6):969–77.

8. Carr J, Nelson J, Wong N, et al. Calcified coronary artery plaque measurement with cardiac CT in population-based studies: standardized protocol of Multi-Ethnic Study of Atherosclerosis (MESA) and Coronary Artery Risk Development in Young Adults (CARDIA) study. Radiology 2005;234(1):35–43.

9. Achenbach S, Daniel G. Current role of cardiac computed tomography. Herz 2007;32:97–107.

10. Boxt LM. CT of valvular heart disease. Int J Cardiovasc Imaging 2005;21(1):105–13.

11. Chen JJ, Jeudy J, Thorn EM, et al. Computed tomography assessment of valvular morphology, function, and disease. J Cardiovasc Comput Tomogr 2009;3(1 Suppl):S47–56.

12. Chen JJ, Manning MA, Frazier AA, et al. CT angiography of the cardiac valves: normal, diseased, and postoperative appearances. Radiographics 2009;29(5):1393–412.

13. Gopalan D, Raj V, Hoey ET. Cardiac CT: noncoronary applications. Postgrad Med J 2010;86(1013):165–73.

14. Chheda SV, Srichai MB, Donnino R, et al. Evaluation of the mitral and aortic valves with cardiac CT angiography. J Thorac Imaging 2010;25(1):76–85.

15. Newland JA, Tamuno P, Pasupati S, et al. Emerging role of MDCT in planning complex structural transcatheter intervention. JACC Cardiovasc Imaging 2014;7(6):627–31.

16. Van Mieghem NM, Piazza N, Anderson RH, et al. Anatomy of the mitral valvular complex and its implications for transcatheter interventions for mitral regurgitation. J Am Coll Cardiol 2010;56(8):617–26.

17. Delgado V, Kapadia S, Marsan NA, et al. Multimodality imaging before, during, and after percutaneous mitral valve repair. Heart 2011;97(20):1704–14.

18. Koo HJ, Yang DH, Oh SY, et al. Demonstration of mitral valve prolapse with CT for planning of mitral valve repair. Radiographics 2014;34(6):1537–52.

19. Ewe SH, Klautz RJ, Schalij MJ, et al. Role of computed tomography imaging for transcatheter valvular repair/insertion. Int J Cardiovasc Imaging 2011;27(8):1179–93.

20. Leipsic J, Wood D, Manders D, et al. The evolving role of MDCT in transcatheter aortic valve replacement: a radiologists' perspective. AJR Am J Roentgenol 2009;193(3):W214–9.

21. Piazza N, Lange R, Martucci G, et al. Patient selection for transcatheter aortic valve implantation: patient risk profile and anatomical selection criteria. Arch Cardiovasc Dis 2012;105(3):165–73.

22. Apfaltrer P, Henzler T, Blanke P, et al. Computed tomography for planning transcatheter aortic valve replacement. J Thorac Imaging 2013;28(4):231–9.

23. Blanke P, Schoepf UJ, Leipsic JA. CT in transcatheter aortic valve replacement. Radiology 2013;269(3):650–69.

24. Ruiz CE, Jelnin V, Kronzon I, et al. Clinical outcomes in patients undergoing percutaneous closure of periprosthetic paravalvular leaks. J Am Coll Cardiol 2011;58(21):2210–7.

25. Ruiz C, Cohen H, Del Valle-Fernandez R, et al. Closure of prosthetic paravalvular leaks: a long way to go. Eur Heart J Suppl 2010;12(Suppl E):E52–62.

26. Kumar R, Jelnin V, Kliger C, et al. Percutaneous paravalvular leak closure. Cardiol Clin 2013;31(3):431–40.

27. Kliger C, Jelnin V, Sharma S, et al. CT angiography-fluoroscopy fusion imaging for percutaneous transapical access. JACC Cardiovasc Imaging 2014;7(2):169–77.

28. Kliger C, Angulo R, Maranan L, et al. Percutaneous complete repair of failed mitral valve prosthesis: simultaneous closure of mitral paravalvular leaks and transcatheter mitral valve implantation - single-centre experience. EuroIntervention 2015;10(11):1336–45.

29. Garcia MJ. NonInvasive cardiovascular imaging: a multimodality approach. Philadelphia: Lippincott Williams & Wilkins; 2012. p. 545.

Mitral Paravalvular Leak Closure

Paul Sorajja, MD

KEYWORDS

- Paravalvular • Leak closure • Regurgitation • Mitral

KEY POINTS

- With appropriate patient selection and operator expertise, percutaneous repair is an established therapy for patients with paravalvular mitral prosthetic regurgitation.
- Percutaneous repair can improve symptoms of heart failure and hemolysis while avoiding the need for repeat sternotomy.
- The procedure should be performed as part of a comprehensive, multidisciplinary valve program with close collaboration between experienced operators and imaging specialists.

Paravalvular regurgitation frequently affects surgical valves in the mitral position, occurring in 5% to 15% of these patients.[1] These patients represent the most common type of paravalvular regurgitation that requires repair, either for treatment of symptoms of heart failure or hemolytic anemia. Although the traditional treatment has been open surgery, percutaneous treatment is the preferred therapy for symptomatic patients.[2] Open surgery carries the risk of reoperation and may not be successful because of poor quality of the underlying tissue. Moreover, the reversible nature of the catheter-based techniques, in the event of an unsuccessful outcome, permits a subsequent surgical attempt if desired. Thus, percutaneous therapy is inherently attractive as a relatively less invasive option for many patients with paravalvular mitral prosthetic regurgitation.

CLINICAL EVALUATION AND PATIENT SELECTION

Patients who may be considered for percutaneous repair require a comprehensive, multidisciplinary evaluation with a heart team approach, whereby there is close collaboration between the cardiologist, interventionalist,

cardiac surgeon, and imaging specialists.[2] Assessment of surgical risk with stratification tools and consultation should be considered, as repeat surgery will not be prohibitive in many patients even though the reoperative risk will be increased relative to the initial surgery.[2–4] All patients with paravalvular prosthetic regurgitation should be evaluated for both hemolytic anemia and active endocarditis, even when there are not suspicious clinical findings. Hemolytic anemia, when present, necessitates a high degree of closure (ideally complete) and should be known when discussing therapeutic options. Active endocarditis is a contraindication to placement of device occluders.

Echocardiography is the primary imaging modality for the evaluation of paravalvular mitral regurgitation. Although 2-dimensional echocardiography is widely used as the initial screening tool, 3-dimensional studies are essential in these patients. Three-dimensional echocardiography provides detailed morphology that is used to plan percutaneous repair, including location, size, and shape of the defects (Fig. 1).[5] In some patients, acoustic shadowing can pose significant challenges for visualizing paravalvular regurgitation. As an additional noninvasive imaging method, cardiac computed tomography

Center for Valve and Structural Heart Disease, Minneapolis Heart Institute, Abbott Northwestern Hospital, 920 East 28th Street, Minneapolis, MN 55407, USA
E-mail address: paul.sorajja@allina.com

Intervent Cardiol Clin 5 (2016) 45–54
http://dx.doi.org/10.1016/j.iccl.2015.08.004

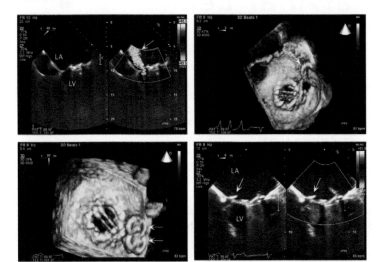

Fig. 1. Echocardiographic imaging of paravalvular regurgitation. Transesophageal echocardiography is essential for assessment of mitral paravalvular regurgitation. Top left: Medial, paravalvular regurgitation of a bileaflet mechanical prosthesis (*arrow*). Top right: Three-dimensional imaging showing the defect and guidance of the steerable catheter (*arrow*). Bottom left: Placement of 2 AVP-vascular plugs (*arrows*). Bottom right: Resolution of the paravalvular regurgitation (*arrow*). LA, left atrium; LV, left ventricle.

(CT) can be useful, as the spatial resolution is not limited by imaging planes. Cardiac CT with contrast can provide information not only on the diagnosis of paravalvular leaks but also their size, orientation, and surrounding calcification. These imaging studies also provide information regarding camera setup in the catheterization laboratory. In some laboratories, cardiac CT is used with fusion imaging to guide the procedure and enhance the success of percutaneous closure (see Computed Tomography Guidance section later).

The imaging examination is performed to determine the location and severity of the paravalvular regurgitation (including size and distance of the defect from the prosthesis annulus), the state of the left and right ventricles, presence of indications for open surgery, and to exclude significant valvular insufficiency. Of note, although echocardiographic quantitation of valvular regurgitation is established, the criteria for severity of paravalvular prosthetic regurgitation are much less studied.[6–8] Moreover, patients with paravalvular mitral regurgitation often have symptoms out of proportion to conventional standards for severity of valvular regurgitation. For symptomatic patients with inconclusive noninvasive studies, strong consideration should be given to evaluation in the cardiac catheterization laboratory with a detailed invasive hemodynamic assessment and left ventriculography (Fig. 2). It is important to note that defects that are not echocardiographically severe can still be hemodynamically significant

and may benefit from therapy; thus, direct examination of dynamic filling pressures may be beneficial. Nonetheless, clinical judgment regarding the severity of these lesions and the likelihood of associated symptoms must be exercised, with the decision to pursue such treatment individualized for all patients.

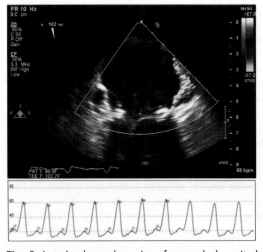

Fig. 2. Invasive hemodynamics of paravalvular mitral prosthetic regurgitation. In this patient, transesophageal imaging shows paravalvular mitral regurgitation that does not fulfill conventional criteria for severity (*top*). However, direct measurement of left atrial pressure shows a mean gradient of 38 mm Hg. Following closure of the paravalvular lesion, there was resolution of the patient's symptoms.

In the 2014 American College of Cardiology Foundation/American Heart Association's practice guidelines on valvular heart disease, percutaneous repair of paravalvular prosthetic regurgitation is recommended for high-risk surgical patients with severe symptoms or hemolysis, who have suitable anatomic features, and when performed in an experienced center (class IIa recommendation).[2] Performance in centers with expertise in the procedure is advised to considerable complexity of the procedure and the relatively infrequent nature of the therapy. Patients with active endocarditis, a rocking prosthesis, significant valvular regurgitation, or paravalvular regurgitation involving a substantial amount of the prosthesis (eg, more than one-third of the annular circumference) should not be treated with percutaneous repair.

TECHNIQUES FOR PERCUTANEOUS REPAIR

Device Occluders and Catheters

Although percutaneous repair of paravalvular regurgitation was first reported more than 2 decades ago, there still remain no devices that are purpose-built for this procedure. Nonetheless, several commercially available ones can be used successfully for the procedure. The most commonly used devices are from the Amplatzer vascular plug family, namely, the AVP-2, AVP-3, and AVP-4 (St. Jude Medical, Fridley, MN). These self-expanding, nitinol devices are deliverable through small-caliber catheters (eg, 4F) and have retention disks to foster stability within the lesion and help reduce the risk of embolization. Although the AVP-2 and AVP-4 devices are used in the United States, the AVP-3 is available only in Europe. The Amplatzer ductal occluders and muscular ventricular septal defect occluders also have been used for percutaneous repair of paravalvular regurgitation, though use of the latter has been anecdotally associated with worsening of hemolysis. Both the ductal and muscular ventricular septal defect occluders also require relatively larger sheaths for delivery but have been successfully used in select cases.

Although the internal diameters of various guide catheters may be described in the manufacturers' labeling, the descriptions often are not consistent in terms of their ability to accommodate the various sizes of the off-label devices. The authors' favored delivery catheter is the Cook Flexor Shuttle sheath (Cook Medical, Bloomington, IN), which comes in a range of sizes suitable for the procedure (most commonly, 4–8F). The Cook sheaths have relatively large internal diameters, which allow simultaneous accommodation of an extrastiff wire and a device occluder. This ability, described as the anchor wire technique, saves invaluable time in the event that the occluder is not suitable for the defect and needs to be replaced, as the anchor wire obviates rewiring the lesion. A 6F Cook Flexor Shuttle will accommodate a 12-mm AVP-2 and a 0.035-in extrastiff Amplatz wire simultaneously (see section on anchor wire technique later). A 4F Cook Flexor Shuttle sheath will facilitate delivery up to an 8-mm AVP-2. Otherwise, a 6F multipurpose guide catheter (Cordis Co, Bridgewater, NJ) can be used to place a 12-mm AVP-2 plug, and a 4F diagnostic multipurpose catheter will accommodate a 4-mm AVP-4.

Technical Approaches

For patients with mitral paravalvular regurgitation, percutaneous repair is usually performed with general anesthesia and transesophageal echocardiography. Intracardiac echocardiography may be considered, but the 3-dimensional imaging from transesophageal echocardiography greatly facilitates the procedure. The most commonly used approach is femoral venous access with transseptal puncture and antegrade cannulation of the defects from the left atrium. In this approach, a 20F DrySeal (W. L. Gore, Flagstaff, AZ) sheath is recommended. This sheath has a balloon inflatable cuff that facilitates hemostasis if multiple wires (anchor or sequential) and delivery catheters are simultaneously used. Other approaches are a direct transapical puncture, with or without guidance from CT, or a retrograde approach via the femoral artery. These two techniques take advantage of the direction of the regurgitant jet with retrograde cannulation from the left ventricle, though these special techniques require considerable expertise to be successful.[9]

For access into the left atrium with the antegrade approach, standard transseptal techniques with guidance from fluoroscopy and echocardiography can be used in most patients. In those with a medial or posterior defect, the acute angulation can pose technical challenges for wiring and catheter advancement. For these patients, a posterior or superior position for the transseptal puncture to gain height on the mitral valve can be beneficial. The atrial septum is usually dilated over a stiff wire with a large dilator (eg, 14F or 16F), followed by placement of the DrySeal sheath in the femoral vein.

A steerable guide (8.5F Agilis catheter, St. Jude, Fridley, MN) is placed into left atrium over the same stiff wire. The guide catheter has a bidirectional tip for anterior-posterior movements and can be rotated in its entirety for medial (ie, counterclockwise) or lateral (ie, clockwise) orientation. The guide catheter has several sizes with medium-curved being the most commonly used; small-curved guides are particularly helpful for medial or posterior defects. A telescoped catheter system, which consists of a 6F 100-cm multipurpose guide and a 5F 125-cm multipurpose diagnostic catheter, is placed into the guide (**Fig. 3**). This coaxial system can then be steered toward the paravalvular defect, which is crossed with the angled-tip, exchange-length Glidewire (Terumo Medical Corporation, Somerset, NJ).

To facilitate crossing, the image intensifier should be placed primarily with orientation of the prosthesis perpendicular to its en face view. Three-dimensional echocardiography or, for those laboratories with biplane capability, imaging with an additional image intensifier is used to orient positioning of the guide anterior/posterior and medial/lateral to the prosthesis. Guidance from comprehensive echocardiography is essential to procedural success, with heavy reliance on constant, clear communication between the imager and interventionalist.

A clock-face approach has been described for this communication. Notably, this approach can be challenging because of the opposite

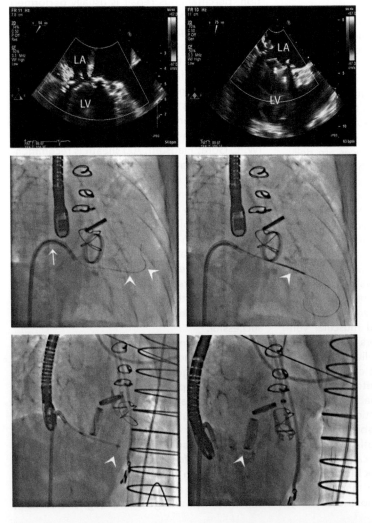

Fig. 3. Percutaneous repair of paravalvular mitral prosthetic regurgitation. Top left: Severe, medial paravalvular mitral prosthetic regurgitation is present on transesophageal echocardiography. Middle left: A steerable sheath (8.5F, St. Jude Agilis catheter) is placed in the left atrium with transseptal puncture (*arrow*) and steered toward the defect, which is then crossed with the wire (*arrowheads*). Middle right: Multipurpose catheters are advanced into the left ventricle (*arrowhead*). Bottom left: The distal disk of a 12-mm AVP-2 plug is extruded into the left ventricle (*arrowhead*). Bottom right: The AVP-2 plug is then positioned and deployed across the paravalvular defect (*arrowhead*). Top right: Mild paravalvular regurgitation is present after deployment of the plug. LA, left atrium; LV, left ventricle.

viewpoints of fluoroscopy versus the surgical view obtained from transesophageal echocardiography. The authors' preferred method is to use anatomically correct terminology (anterior vs posterior, lateral vs medial), with triangulation between the aortic valve (ie, anterior), left atrial appendage (ie, anterolateral), and atrial septum (ie, medial).[10] For patients with mechanical valves, describing the location defect relative to the prosthetic commissures can also assist with orientation of the steerable guide system.

Once the defect has been crossed, fluoroscopy must demonstrate positioning of the guidewires external to the prosthesis ring. The two multipurpose catheters are placed sequentially into the left ventricle, followed by removal of the diagnostic catheter (see Fig. 3). At this point, one may choose to deliver a device occluder through the 6F guide, which can accommodate a 12-mm AVP-2 vascular plug. Alternatively, the entire coaxial system can be exchanged over a 0.032-in extrastiff Amplatz wire for a larger catheter (eg, 90-cm, 6F–8F Cook Flexor Shuttle) that will enable either multiple device placements or anchor wire techniques. In some instances, the location of the defect (eg, medial) or its pathologic qualities (eg, calcification, serpiginous) may not permit placement of the Cook sheath with an 0.032-in Amplatz wire alone, and a transcatheter heart rail is required (see later discussion).

Following placement of the delivery sheath, the distal retention disk of the occluder is extruded from the guide into the left ventricle and the defect is then straddled with the retention disks on both sides (see Fig. 3). At this point, it is essential to exclude leaflet impingement on both echocardiography and fluoroscopy with release of tension on the delivery cable. Leaflet impingement is much more common with mechanical prostheses and stentless bioprostheses. Anterior-superior defects are particularly prone to movement of the device occluder following release. Once significant reduction in the regurgitation has occurred without prosthetic leaflet impingement, the device occluder is fully decoupled from the delivery cable.

In the retrograde approach from the femoral artery, a coronary catheter (eg, Judkins right, Amplatz left or right, or internal mammary) is placed into the left ventricle and oriented posterior toward the defect. The femoral retrograde technique can be considered when the transseptal approach is not successful, especially for the

treatment of medial defects. Use of relatively softer wires, such as 0.014-in or 0.018-in coronary guidewires, is recommended as the relatively greater stiffness of the Glidewire often reduces steerability of the coronary catheter. The coronary guidewire is snared in the left atrium for creation of a rail, and a 4F Cook Sheath with a 0.018-in internal diameter can then be used to exchange for a stiffer wire. In the transapical technique, cannulation of the defect and device placement is similar to the antegrade approach. CT guidance has also been demonstrated to be beneficial when performing the apical puncture and for steering toward the paravalvular defect (see section on CT guidance later).

Transcatheter Rails

Placement of delivery catheters can be challenging because of the underlying tissue pathology, which may lead to the development of serpiginous and calcific defects. In these instances, transcatheter rails provide greater support for their passage, especially when large sheaths are required.

Transcatheter rails were originally described for the treatment of congenital heart lesions. Following placement of a guidewire across the paravalvular defect, the wire is snared and then exteriorized to provide the operator with both ends of the wire and greater support for delivery catheter placement. The rail also serves as an anchor to enable the operator to recross the defect in the event different device occluders are required. These rails are used for the treatment of all types of paravalvular lesions. For patients with mitral paravalvular defects, the transcatheter rail can be placed in the left atrial-ventricular-aortic or left atrial-ventricular-apical position (Fig. 4). Once the rail has been created, the operator can advance a guide catheter with support from an assistant who provides tension on both ends of the wire.

When using transcatheter rails, it is important to note that injury to surrounding structures can easily occur. Harm can result from tension on the guidewire and can arise from damage to the prosthetic leaflets, native aortic valve, severe bradycardia from pressure on the atrioventricular node, myocardial injury, and, if present, disruption of the mitral valve apparatus from chordal entanglement. Thus, transcatheter heart rails should only be performed by experienced operators and with careful hemodynamic monitoring and simultaneous echocardiography.

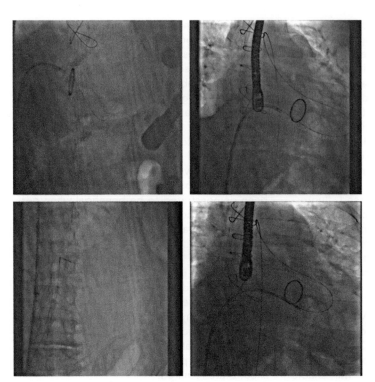

Fig. 4. Creation of a transcatheter rail. Top left: The defect is wired with a Glidewire antegrade from the left atrium. Top right: The wire is passed through the aortic valve into the descending aorta for snaring. Bottom left: The wire is snared with a 15-mm gooseneck and exteriorized. Bottom right: Over this rail, tension on both ends of the wire facilitates passage of an 8F Cook Flexor Shuttle across the paravalvular defect followed by placement of a 12-mm AVP-2 vascular plug.

Multiple Device Placement and Anchor Wiring

Paravalvular defects are frequently eccentric and reside close to the surgical sewing ring. As a result, successful closure can be challenging with the use of large occluders, as device overhang can result in leaflet impingement. In these instances, multiple smaller device occluders can be placed to reduce device overhang. In this technique, a large-bore guide catheter (eg, ≥6F Cook Flexor Shuttle) is placed into the ventricle once the defect is crossed with a hydrophilic guidewire. The guide catheter facilitates placement of multiple, extrastiff guidewires; these wires can then be used to place the delivery catheters either simultaneously or sequentially over each wire. In the simultaneous approach, two 0.032-in extrastiff Amplatz wires can be advanced through the sheath into the left ventricle, followed by placement of 2 multipurpose guides that have been telescoped individually over diagnostic multipurpose catheters (Fig. 5).

The authors' favored approach is to place the device occluders sequentially, leaving an anchor wire behind during the placement of each plug (Fig. 6). In this technique, the operator deploys a device occluder across the paravalvular defect with a 0.032-in extrastiff wire alongside in the left ventricle (ie, the anchor). The delivery sheath is removed and then reinserted with a dilator over the 0.032-in anchor wire only, leaving the delivery cable that is coupled to the device occluder exterior to the sheath. Another device occluder can then be inserted with the anchor wire in place, and the process may be repeated as necessary for treatment of the entire lesion. When anticipating placement of only a single device, the anchor wire technique is also useful for maintaining a position across the paravalvular defect if an occluder needs to be exchanged for different or multiple other devices. The aforementioned transcatheter rail technique can also be used an anchor wire. In the anchor wire technique, a large-bore vascular sheath is required to accommodate the multiple delivery catheters and wires either from the femoral venous or arterial access point. The 12F to 26F DrySeal sheath, with its inflatable cuff, is uniquely suitable for maintaining hemostasis for this purpose.

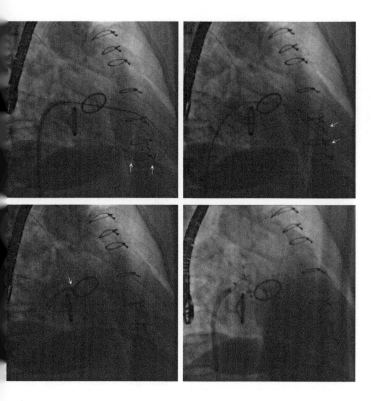

Fig. 5. Simultaneous deployment of device occluders. Top left: Following placement of a 6F multipurpose guide in the left ventricle, two 0.032-n extrastiff Amplatz wires are placed (arrows). Top right: Over these 2 wires, separate telescoped multipurpose catheters (5F and 6F) are advanced into the left ventricle. The diagnostic catheters are removed, followed by extrusion of the distal disks of two 12-mm AVP-2 plugs (arrows). Bottom left: The plugs and multipurpose catheters are withdrawn together to straddle the device occluders across the single defect (arrow). Bottom right: The plugs are deployed and decoupled from the delivery catheters.

Computed Tomography Guidance

Cardiac CT easily identifies the site of paravalvular regurgitation and can assist with planning of the procedure. CT imaging helps with sizing of the defect, provides information on its course and surrounding calcification, and helps to exclude the presence of valvular regurgitation. The last capability may be of particular clinical benefit when there is significant acoustic shadowing on echocardiography. Imaging with electrocardiogram gating is performed with contrast, a slice thickness of 0.5 or 0.6 mm for maximal spatial resolution, and 3 or more reconstruction intervals to identify the defect. The imager examines data from echocardiography, and the CT scan is reconstructed with views of the exit point of the regurgitant jet, whose paravalvular continuity can then be examined. In some laboratories, the fusion imaging with CT overlay during fluoroscopy is used during the procedure to facilitate transapical access, cannulation of the defect, and device placement. This approach has been well described by experienced operators to increase procedural efficiency and success.[11]

CLINICAL OUTCOMES

Although percutaneous repair of paravalvular regurgitation was first described more than 25 years ago, most of the development of this therapy has been in the past 8 years.[12–14] Procedural success, using a strict definition of reduction to mild regurgitation or less with no major adverse events, occurs in approximately 80% of patients (~90% for moderate residual regurgitation or less).[13,14] Complications are relatively infrequent. In a series of 115 patients, the 30-day rates of adverse events were 2.6% for stroke, 0.9% for emergency surgery, 1.7% for sudden or unexplained death, and 5.2% for periprocedural bleeding. Periprocedural bleeding can arise from cardiac perforation, particularly with apical puncture, as well as use of large vascular access sheaths.[15] Care must be exercised bridging anticoagulation. Of note, closure of apical puncture sites with vascular plugs or surgical glue has been used to help promote hemostasis of these sites. In the 2 largest series combined, device embolization occurred in 4 (or 2.5%) of 159 patients. The AVP-2 and AVP-4 plugs are particularly easy to retrieve through

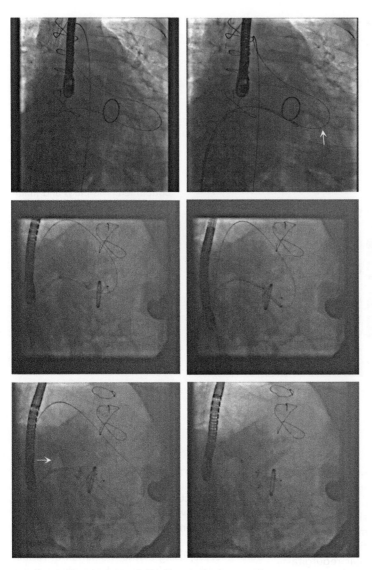

Fig. 6. Anchor wire technique with transcatheter rail. Following creation of a transcatheter rail (*top left*), an 8F Cook Flexor Shuttle sheath is placed into the left ventricle and a 12-mm AVP-2 plug is extruded along side the rail (*arrow, top right*). The AVP-2 plug is deployed across the defect, followed by removal of the delivery sheath is removed (*middle left*). The delivery sheath is then reinserted over the rail only, leaving the delivery cable still coupled to the AVP-2 plug. A second 12-mm AVP-2 plug is then extruded alongside the rail and first AVP-2 plug (*middle right*). The second AVP-2 plug is placed across the defect while the first plug is still coupled to the delivery cable (*arrow, bottom left*). If desired, the maneuver of removing and reinserting the sheath over only the rail can be repeated to place additional devices. In this instance, adequate closure was achieved with the 2 AVP-2 plugs, which were then deployed (*bottom right*).

snaring techniques in the periphery vasculature. Procedural death is uncommon (~0.5%) despite the complexity of the techniques.

The most common reasons for procedural failure are prosthetic leaflet impingement and the inability to cross the defects of the wire or delivery catheter. Leaflet impingement can occur with any prosthesis (~5% of cases) but is more common in mechanical valves because of the absence of struts. Impingement can be minimized through the use of multiple smaller devices, though the circular shape of these occluders and close proximity of the defect to the surgical annular ring can still be difficult.

Before device release, particular care must be taken to ensure proper leaflet function for both bioprosthetic and mechanical valves with release of tension, using both imaging and hemodynamic assessments with gradient calculation to be performed. Because the release of tension on the system after device release can lead to repositioning of the occluder, the possibility of leaflet impingement should be reassessed after final deployment.

Clinical success and relief of symptoms are related to the degree of residual regurgitation and are greater for patients with symptoms of heart failure than for those with hemolysis.[16]

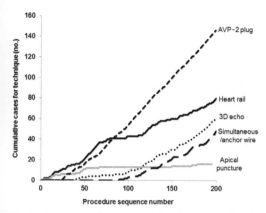

Fig. 7. Adoption of imaging and catheter-based techniques with increasing operator experience in percutaneous repair of paravalvular prosthetic regurgitation. The graph shows the cumulative number of times a technique was used over an experience of 200 patients. 3D, 3 dimensional. (*From* Sorajja P, Cabalka AK, Hagler DJ, et al. The learning curve in percutaneous repair of paravalvular prosthetic regurgitation: an analysis of 200 cases. JACC Cardiovasc Interv 2014;7:527; with permission.)

Successful treatment of hemolysis requires a relatively greater degree of closure (ideally complete). Operator experience with the adoption of recently evolved techniques (eg, anchor wire, 3-dimension imaging, transcatheter rails) is an important predictor of success with the therapy (Fig. 7).[17]

In a long-term evaluation of 126 patients who underwent percutaneous repair of paravalvular prosthetic regurgitation (aged 67 ±13 years; Society of Thoracic Surgeons Predicted Risk of Mortality, 6.7 ± 5.4%), the 3-year survival was 64% (Fig. 8).[16] Cardiac death occurred in 9.5%; the incidence of noncardiac death was between 7.1% and 12.7%, owing to the significant morbidity of these patients. Notably, 72% of the survivors were free of severe symptoms or need for open cardiac surgery. Also of note, New York Heart Association functional class improved only in those patients with residual regurgitation of mild or less.

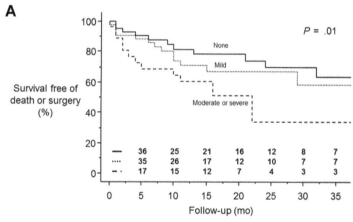

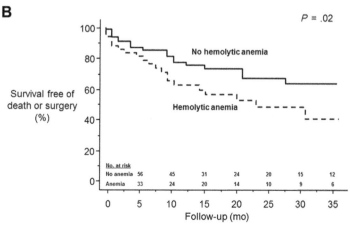

Fig. 8. Survival after percutaneous repair of paravalvular prosthetic regurgitation. (*A*) Survival free of death or need for cardiac surgery according to residual regurgitation after paravalvular repair. (*B*) Survival free of death or need for cardiac surgery according to the presence of hemolytic anemia as an indication for the procedure. (*From* Sorajja P, Cabalka AK, Hagler DJ, et al. Long-term follow-up of percutaneous repair of paravalvular prosthetic regurgitation. J Am Coll Cardiol 2011;58:2222; with permission.)

SUMMARY

With appropriate patient selection and operator expertise, percutaneous repair is an established therapy for patients with paravalvular mitral prosthetic regurgitation. Percutaneous repair can improve symptoms of heart failure and hemolysis while avoiding the need for repeat sternotomy. The procedure should be performed as part of a comprehensive, multidisciplinary valve program with close collaboration between experienced operators and imaging specialists.

REFERENCES

1. Davila-Roman VG, Waggoner AD, Kennard ED, et al. Prevalence and severity of paravalvular regurgitation in the Artificial Valve Endocarditis Reduction Trial (AVERT) echocardiography study. J Am Coll Cardiol 2004;44:1467–72.
2. Nishimura RA, Otto CM, Bonow RO, et al. 2014 AHA/ACC guideline for the management of patients with valvular heart disease: a report of the American College of Cardiology/American Heart Association task force on practice guidelines. J Am Coll Cardiol 2014;63:e57–185.
3. Maganti M, Rao V, Armstrong S, et al. Redo valvular surgery in elderly patients. Ann Thorac Surg 2009; 87:521–5.
4. Luciani N, Nasso G, Anselmi A, et al. Repeat valvular operations: bench optimization of conventional surgery. Ann Thorac Surg 2006;81:1279–83.
5. Altiok E, Frick M, Meyer CG, et al. Comparison of two- and three-dimensional transthoracic echocardiography to cardiac magnetic resonance imaging for assessment of paravalvular regurgitation after transcatheter aortic valve implantation. Am J Cardiol 2014;113:1859–66.
6. Zoghbi WA, Enriquez-Sarano M, Foster E, et al. Recommendations for evaluation of the severity of native valvular regurgitation with two-dimensional and Doppler echocardiography. J Am Soc Echocardiogr 2003;16:777–802.
7. Kappetein AP, Head SJ, Genereux P, et al. Updated standardized endpoint definitions for transcatheter aortic valve implantation: the Valve Academic Research Consortium-2 consensus document. J Am Coll Cardiol 2012; 60:1438–54.
8. Zogbhi WA, Chambers JB, Dumesnil JG, et al. Recommendations for evaluation of prosthetic valves with echocardiography and Doppler ultrasound. J Am Soc Echocardiogr 2009;22: 975–1014.
9. Jelnin V, Dudly Y, Einhorn BN, et al. Clinical experience with percutaneous left ventricular transapical access for interventions in structural heart defects a safe access and secure exit. JACC Cardiovasc Interv 2011;4:868–74.
10. Spoon DB, Malouf JF, Spoon JN, et al. Mitral paravalvular leak: description and assessment of a novel anatomical method of localization. JACC Cardiovasc Imaging 2013;6:1212–4.
11. Kliger C, Jelnin V, Sharma S, et al. CT angiography-fluoroscopy fusion imaging for percutaneous transpical access. JACC Cardiovasc Imaging 2014;7: 169–77.
12. Hourihan M, Perry SB, Mandell VS, et al. Transcatheter closure of valvular and perivalvular leaks. J Am Coll Cardiol 1992;20:1371–7.
13. Ruiz CE, Jelnin V, Kronzon I, et al. Clinical outcomes in patients undergoing percutaneous closure of periprosthetic paravalvular leaks. J Am Coll Cardiol 2011;58:2210–7.
14. Sorajja P, Cabalka AK, Hagler DJ, et al. Percutaneous repair of paravalvular prosthetic regurgitation: acute and 30-day outcomes in 115 patients. Circ Cardiovasc Interv 2011;4:314–21.
15. Pitta SR, Cabalka AK, Rihal CS. Complications associated with left ventricular puncture. Catheter Cardiovasc Interv 2010;76:993–7.
16. Sorajja P, Cabalka AK, Hagler DJ, et al. Long-term follow-up of percutaneous repair of paravalvular prosthetic regurgitation. J Am Coll Cardiol 2011; 58:2218–24.
17. Sorajja P, Cabalka AK, Hagler DJ, et al. The learning curve in percutaneous repair of paravalvular prosthetic regurgitation: an analysis of 200 cases. JACC Cardiovasc Interv 2014;7:521–9.

Targeted Transseptal Access for MitraClip Percutaneous Mitral Valve Repair

Gagan D. Singh, MD*, Thomas W. Smith, MD, Jason H. Rogers, MD

KEYWORDS

- Percutaneous mitral valve repair • MitraClip • Transseptal • Baylis • BRK • Interatrial septum

KEY POINTS

- Targeted transseptal puncture remains the most critical initial part of the overall MitraClip procedure.
- Care and attention must be implemented for patient safety in choosing the optimal puncture site.
- A consistent and step-by-step methodical approach is recommended.
- As experienced operators are targeting more complex and nontraditional pathologies, use of adjunctive tools and maneuvers (outlined in this review) are paramount to achieving successful targeted transseptal access and ultimately procedural success.

INTRODUCTION

Percutaneous transseptal puncture and access to the left atrium (LA) for diagnostic catheterization has been in use since its description in 1959 by Drs Ross, Braunwald, and Morrow.[1,2] Its use expanded for balloon mitral valvuloplasty and over the past few decades for electrophysiologic procedures.[3] More recently, there has been a relative explosion of structural heart interventions from the LA (eg, percutaneous mitral valve repair with MitraClip (Abbott Vascular, Menlo Park, California, USA), percutaneous left atrial appendage ligation/closure with the Lariat [SentreHEART, Redwood City, CA, USA] or Watchman device [Boston Scientific, Marlborough, MA, USA]) also necessitating transseptal puncture.[4] However, for the latter interventions, precision of the transseptal puncture is paramount, as an off-target transseptal puncture can easily add significant complexity and time to the procedure. The purpose of this review is

to provide the rationale, septal anatomy, and tools available to achieve successful targeted transseptal puncture for the MitraClip procedure with a few special scenarios whereby targeted transseptal puncture can still be achieved.

ROLE OF TARGETED TRANSSEPTAL PUNCTURE FOR MITRACLIP

Targeted transseptal puncture is the initial crucial part of the MitraClip procedure. It determines the height and position of the guiding catheter relative to the coaptation plane of the mitral leaflets and influences the degrees of freedom available for the clip delivery system (CDS) and guiding catheter to maneuver. Adequate range of movement of the CDS and guide is required to successfully deliver the MitraClip and grasp the leaflets. A poorly positioned transseptal puncture will result in difficulty maneuvering the device in the LA. The guide may be inappropriately close to important

Division of Cardiovascular Medicine, University of California Davis Medical Center, 4860 Y Street, Suite 2820, Sacramento, CA 95817, USA
* Corresponding author.
E-mail address: drsingh@ucdavis.edu

Intervent Cardiol Clin 5 (2016) 55–69
http://dx.doi.org/10.1016/j.iccl.2015.08.005
2211-7458/16/$ – see front matter

structures, such as the aorta by puncturing anterosuperiorly, or the guide may be directed toward the posterior wall of the LA by an inappropriately inferoposterior puncture. The puncture may be too high above the valve coaptation plane, leaving insufficient height for the CDS and clip to reach and grasp the leaflets. Finally, the puncture may be too low, making it difficult to retract the CDS and grasp the leaflets. Ultimately, a suboptimal transseptal puncture site limits the range of movement that is built into the MitraClip system and may result in inadequate treatment of underlying mitral regurgitation etiology.

INTERATRIAL SEPTAL ANATOMY AND RELATIONSHIP TO ADJACENT STRUCTURES

Successful transseptal puncture mandates a 3-dimensional (3D) understanding of the interatrial septal/fossa anatomy and its relationship to the surrounding structures. Failure to understand the overall spatial anatomy will lead to difficulty in appropriately maneuvering the tools needed for successful targeted transseptal puncture.

Under most normal anatomic conditions, the right atrium (RA) lies anterior to the LA. Furthermore, the interatrial septum is not in an exact midcoronal plane; rather, it lies off axis with the septum proceeding from the patients' left to the right in the anteroposterior direction (Fig. 1). This natural orientation of the interatrial septum is the rationale for having the initial position of the transseptal needle at the 4- or 5-o'clock position (see step-by-step instructions later) so the needle (and the tent) is perpendicular to the fossa. For purposes of transseptal puncture, the interatrial septum is initially visualized on transesophageal echo (TEE) in a superior-inferior view (ie, bicaval view) in which both the superior vena cava (SVC) and the inferior vena cava (IVC) are aligned in conjunction with the interatrial septum (Fig. 2, top left inset). When the bicaval plane is further assessed with both the mitral and tricuspid valves en face in a reconstructed CT, the relationship between a superior puncture and the mitral valve becomes evident (Fig. 3). An inferior puncture would move the delivery system far posterior in relation to the mitral valve making clip delivery challenging (particularly for more lateral jets). The second view used is the short-axis view in which the interatrial fossa is viewed in the anteroposterior projection with the aortic valve and the posterior wall aligned in conjunction with the interatrial septum (see Fig. 2, top right inset). It is important to appreciate that the bicaval and the short-axis views are not perpendicular to each other. Rather the short axis is often obtained with the omniplane of the TEE probe rotated to 30° to 60°. In the short-axis view, rotation of the transseptal needle clockwise not only moves the intended puncture site away from the aorta but also allows the puncture site to move away from the mitral annular plane, allowing one to gain transseptal height. This concept is best appreciated in the 3D reconstruction of a 4-chamber view (Fig. 4).

EQUIPMENT

For MitraClip delivery, transseptal puncture can be performed safely under the guidance of

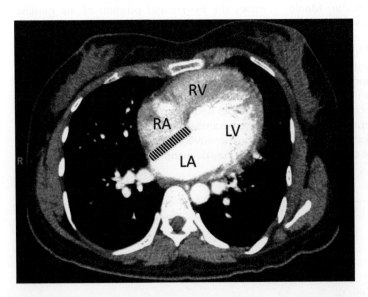

Fig. 1. Computed tomography of the chest. Axial view at the level of the heart, which demonstrates the relative anterior position of the RA to the LA. The interatrial septum (black-yellow shaded region) is not parallel to the midcoronal plane and rather is off axis with the septum directed from the patient's left to their right in the anteroposterior direction. LV, left ventricle; RV, right ventricle.

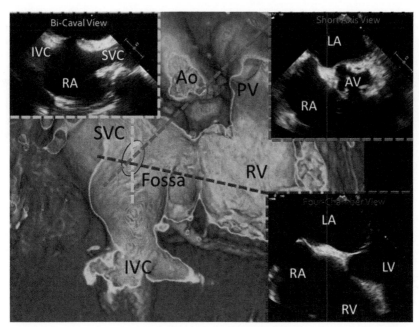

Fig. 2. Reconstructed computed tomography demonstrates spatial anatomy of the interatrial fossa in relation to other right-sided structures. Ao, aorta; AV, *aortic* valve; LV, left ventricle; PV, pulmonic valve; RV, right ventricle.

simultaneous TEE. The traditional catheter and needle combinations include the Mullins sheath, dilator, and standard Brockenbrough (BRK, St. Jude Medical, St Paul, Minnesota, USA) needle (Fig. 5). Other options available commercially consist of the BRK series of transseptal needles and the Swartz™ Braided Transseptal Guiding Introducers SL Series (SL, St. Jude Medical, St Paul, Minnesota, USA) series of transseptal sheaths. In general, the shape of the transseptal sheath has little importance to the curve needed to engage the septum. As long as the needle is located within the

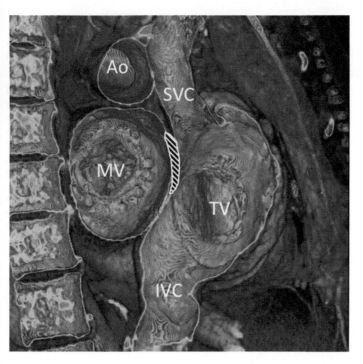

Fig. 3. Reconstructed computed tomography of the chest demonstrates the relationship of the mitral valve (MV, bioprosthetic) and the tricuspid valve (TV) in relationship to the interatrial fossa (black-yellow shaded region). As the transseptal needle is retracted superiorly to inferiorly, the needle moves to the posterior aspect of the MV. This reconstruction highlights the importance of a relatively superior puncture. Ao, aorta.

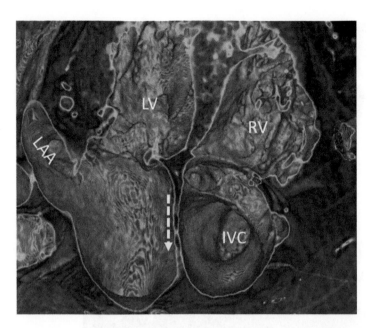

Fig. 4. Three-dimensional reconstruction of computed tomography of the chest depicting a 4-chamber view with the IVC en face. Note that as a transseptal needle is rotated clockwise (*arrow*), the needle moves away from the mitral annular plane, thereby increasing the transseptal height. LAA, LA appendage; LV, left ventricle; RV, right ventricle.

catheter, the catheter will generally take the curve of the needle. It is only after this needle is removed that the catheter will take its intended shape. Once the sheath is in the LA and the needle and dilator are removed, the authors use a 7F multipurpose catheter to direct a stiff 0.035-in guidewire into the left upper pulmonary vein. The Agilis NxT steerable introducers (St. Jude Medical, St Paul, MN) are specialized catheters with adjustable curves that may be particularly suitable for

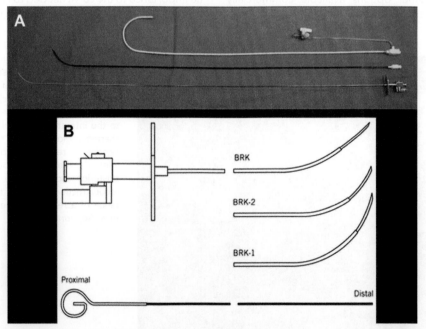

Fig. 5. (A) Components of a transseptal puncture system. From top to bottom: Mullins sheath, dilator, and transseptal needle. (B) Curve options: 2 adult curves (BRK and BRK-1) and 2 pediatric (BRK and BRK-2). Available length: 3 adult (71, 89, 98 cm) and one pediatric (56 cm). The 98-cm needle designed for use with the Agilis NxT steerable introducer (St. Jude Medical, St Paul, MN). (*From* Lasala JM, Rogers JH, editors. Interventional procedures for adult structural heart disease. Philadelphia: Saunders; 2014; with permission.)

complex anatomy. Depending on personal experience, preferences, and anatomy, operators may choose to use specific equipment. Regardless of the equipment chosen, the key to the transseptal procedure lies in clear visualization by TEE and careful selection of the puncture site.

BASIC STEP-BY-STEP TECHNIQUE

After successful venous access, the authors immediately administer 2000 IU of intravenous (IV) heparin to minimize the risk of thrombus formation on the transseptal equipment in the RA before crossing. Next, using a multipurpose A (MPA) catheter, a 0.032-in wire is advanced to the SVC under fluoroscopic guidance. The MPA catheter and the venous sheath are removed over the wire; the transseptal sheath and dilator, such as the Mullins (Medtronic, Minneapolis, Minnesota, USA) or SL-1 sheaths, are advanced into the SVC. Needle and sheath preparation and handling are described in Fig. 6. The wire is then removed, and the transseptal needle is advanced to near the distal tip of the sheath and under fluoroscopic guidance (usually to ~1 cm from the tip of the dilator). The orientation of the needle and sheath

must be maintained by matching the metal arrow on the needle's hub to the direction of sheath's sidearm (Fig. 7). The authors find it is helpful to then move the needle and sheath together with one hand grasping both as a single unit (see Fig. 6E). This technique also maintains a constant and safe needle distance from the tip of the dilator. The sheath, dilator, and needle are oriented such that the system is pointing toward a 4- or 5-o'clock position. As the orientation of the interatrial septum is off axis from the standard midcoronal plane, this particular positioning of the transseptal system allows the needle to be perpendicular to the septum on initial engagement.

Under fluoroscopic and TEE guidance, the sheath and needle are slowly and carefully pulled back to the junction of the SVC and RA. The TEE at this time is focused on the interatrial septum in a dedicated bicaval view (see Fig. 2). On fluoroscopy, most operators may note a 2-step drop or a sudden downward movement of the needle. The first drop occurs as the needle drops from the SVC into the RA (one may note a premature atrial contraction at this point). The next drop occurs as the needle falls into the fossa ovalis from the RA. The operator can often

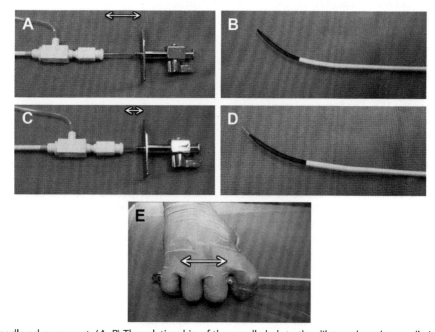

Fig. 6. Needle advancement. (A, B) The relationship of the needle hub to the dilator when the needle is within the transseptal sheath dilator (2-headed arrow). (C, D) The needle is advanced slightly out of the dilator, and the distance between the needle hub and dilator decreases (2-headed arrow). (E) Technique for holding the transseptal system. The entire system is grasped within the hand to allow the system to move as one unit. The sheath and dilator and are grasped with the index finger and thumb, and the needle is grasped with the remaining fingers. This technique ensures a constant relationship between the needle and sheath (2-headed arrow) and avoids inadvertent needle advancement. (From Lasala JM, Rogers JH, editors. Interventional procedures for adult structural heart disease. Philadelphia: Saunders; 2014; with permission.)

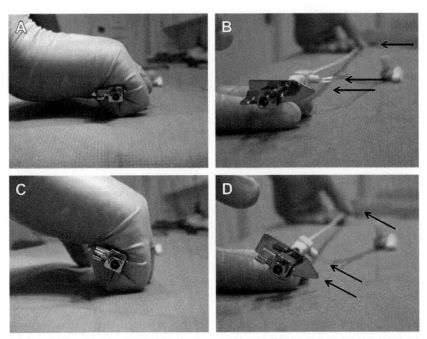

Fig. 7. The transseptal (TS) sheath and needle are moved as one system by rotating the hand. The arrow on the TS needle should be aligned with the sidearm of the sheath, which is oriented toward the curve of the TS sheath (*arrows*). (*A, B*) The system in the horizontal (3 o'clock) position (*arrows*). (*C, D*) The system in the 4-o'clock position (*arrows*), which is the preferred angle of crossing for most structurally normal hearts. Note that this angle will change with RA or LA enlargement. (*From* Lasala JM, Rogers JH, editors. Interventional procedures for adult structural heart disease. Philadelphia: Saunders; 2014; with permission.)

estimate the location of the fossa by the position of the TEE probe, which is focused on the interatrial septum.

At this time, attention is focused almost completely on the TEE. The first view is the bicaval view in which the superior-inferior orientation of the puncture needed is determined. The ideal position in a routine endovascular valve edge-to-edge repair study (EVEREST) II–type patient would be just slightly superior from the midpoint in this view.[5] The sheath dilator should be used to tent the septum. If tenting is not clearly seen in the bicaval view, the dilator is tenting the fossa off axis. The echocardiographer can rotate the TEE probe anteriorly or posteriorly to determine the location, and the interventionalist can make appropriate adjustments to reach the true bicaval plane. Once this position is achieved, the TEE is used to display the short-axis view at the level of the aortic valve (see **Fig. 2**, top right inset). This view provides an anterior-posterior perspective on the transseptal location. To manipulate the transseptal needle and sheath posteriorly, the entire system is torqued clockwise. The ideal position is slightly posterior of the midline. It is important to recognize that if the dilator is tenting the septum too aggressively, clockwise or

counterclockwise torque of the sheath may simply cause the tip of the sheath to pivot at the site of tenting. It may, therefore, be necessary to slightly disengage (pull back) the catheter/needle system from the septum to allow repositioning. The same principle applies when adjusting the sheath in an anteroposterior direction by either advancing or withdrawing the system. Finally, because the fossa ovalis is an elliptical shape, movement of the sheath posteriorly may actually result in a more inferior position, so the operator should check orthogonal TEE views to ensure proper orientation in both planes before puncturing.

The next view is the 4- or 5-chamber view in which the perpendicular (vertical) height of the transseptal tenting from the mitral valve is measured (see **Figs. 2** and **4**). In general, this distance should be between 3.5 and 4.5 cm, although this height may need to be adjusted for nontraditional pathology (eg, commissural mitral regurgitation [MR], large LA, and so forth, discussed later). The mitral valve reference point is either the mitral valve annular plane or the point of coaptation of the mitral valve leaflets (**Fig. 8**). Usually, in patients who have mitral valve prolapse, the mitral annulus is a reasonable guide for height measurements. However, in

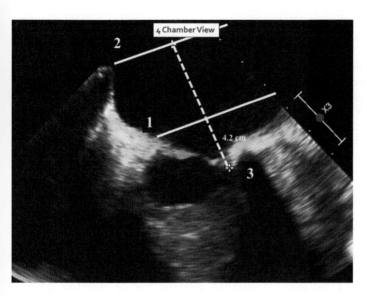

Fig. 8. Height assessment: Once the superoposterior fossa is engaged, then switch to the 4-chamber view. First (1), a horizontal line is drawn on the mitral annular plane. Next (2), an additional line (parallel to the mitral annular plane) is drawn at the site of transseptal tenting (referred to as the transseptal plane). Finally (3), the transseptal height is determined by measuring the distance from the transseptal plane down to the coaptation plane.

patients with functional MR, the point of coaptation is usually lower because of the restricted leaflet mobility. Hence, the authors would recommend using the point of leaflet coaptation in patients with functional MR as a point of reference. Once the suitability of the proposed transseptal puncture site has been confirmed by the views described, puncture across the septum is performed. The transseptal needle is attached to a slow infusion of saline from the manifold. Additionally, transseptal puncture is performed in the short axis of the interatrial septum in efforts to avoid hitting vital structures (eg, posterior atrial wall, aorta, and so forth). Once appropriate positioning is confirmed, the needle is advanced just beyond the tip of the dilator and gentle forward pressure is exerted. Generally, a small pop is felt as the needle traverses the interatrial septum. Once the tip of the needle enters the LA, on fluoroscopy (and simultaneous TEE), a slight forward jump should be noted; bubbles in the LA will be seen (from the slow infusion of saline); and finally as the manifold is then converted to pressure, LA pressure waveforms should be noted. Once transseptal puncture is confirmed, the needle and sheath should be rotated slightly counterclockwise (anterior) to avoid inadvertent puncture of the posterior wall of the LA. The dilator and sheath (as a system) are then advanced over the needle into the LA preferably under TEE guidance. The sheath is then advanced over the needle and dilator; finally the needle and dilator are then carefully removed, and the transseptal sheath is carefully aspirated and flushed to avoid any air entry or thrombus formation and connected to pressure to determine preprocedural LA pressure and waveform.

Once the transseptal puncture is done and the sheath or guide is across the interatrial septum, additional IV heparin is administered to achieve an activated clotting time (ACT) greater than 250 s.

SPECIAL CONSIDERATIONS
Noncentral (Commissural) Mitral Regurgitation

Unlike the classic EVEREST II patient, many patients may have significant pathology arising from the medial aspect (A3/P3), lateral aspect (A1/P1), or commissures of the mitral valve. In the literature, jets from non-EVEREST pathology have been referred to as noncentral MR. The overall prevalence of noncentral MR is unknown. However, as more data from European and US registries becomes available, it is evident that operators are approaching noncentral pathology with increasing frequency.[6,7] Based on the location of the noncentral pathology (medial vs lateral), the target transseptal puncture site can change to aid in clip delivery. The commissural subvalvular apparatus contains a complex structure of fan-shaped chordae, which theoretically increases the risk for subvalvular entanglement with the MitraClip system. However, in the only series evaluating outcomes after MitraClip repair of central versus noncentral MR, there was no difference in procedural outcomes or complications (eg, clip entanglement).[6] Hence, as worldwide experience increases with the MitraClip system, noncentral MR targets will continue to be an important subset of patients encountered by MitraClip operators.

Classically, lower transseptal puncture heights have been endorsed for more medial jets and higher transseptal heights for more lateral jets (**Fig. 9**). This recommendation is in part due to the maneuverability of the guide catheter. For more medial jets, the entire guide catheter can be retracted (sometimes even back into the RA). For more lateral jets, the system is advanced deeper into the LA. As the system is advanced into the LA, transseptal height is gained (**Fig. 10**). Hence, on preprocedural evaluation, if a lateral jet is the primary target, a lower transseptal height may be targeted.

However, it is more than just the transseptal height that is important when targeting noncentral jets. It is important to understand that the relationship between the interatrial septum and the coaptation plane are not perfectly perpendicular (**Fig. 11**). Rather, when the mitral valve is viewed en face in its normal anatomic position in the chest cavity (from the posterior aspect of the heart), the coaptation plane is curvilinear with the more lateral commissure located at the 11-o'clock position and the more medial commissure located at the 5-o'clock position. Hence, when a superior transseptal site is selected, this allows you to easily advance the MitraClip guide catheter toward more lateral and central mitral valve pathology without any need for significant flexion of the guide catheter (**Fig. 12A**). However,

if a medial jet is targeted with a more superior puncture, this will require flexion of the guide catheter and make the approach with the CDS more challenging. This need can be obviated with a more inferior (and posterior) puncture allowing you to directly approach the medial jet without substantial flexion (see **Fig. 12B**). Importantly, the terms *superior* and *inferior* used in this section relate to the position of the transseptal puncture in relation to the SVC and IVC. The position along the bicaval plane has little impact on the overall transseptal height, which is more a relation of the anterior or posterior torque of the transseptal needle (reviewed earlier).

Preexisting Patent Foramen Ovale/Atrial Septal Defect

Anatomically, patent foramen ovale (PFO) is a tunnel-like remnant that is directed superoanteriorly. In general, the authors do not recommend crossing the PFO to enter the LA, as the guide catheter is biased in a trajectory that is unsuitable for the treatment of most mitral valve pathologies (**Fig. 13A, B**). The presence of a PFO may render the remainder of the interatrial septum elastic and may be difficult to provide adequate tenting or anchoring on the intended site of puncture. Even if the intended position is identified, as the needle is advanced for puncture, it may slide off the intended site of puncture because of the laxity of the septum. In cases such as these, the mandrel supplied with the BRK needle can be used to help stick

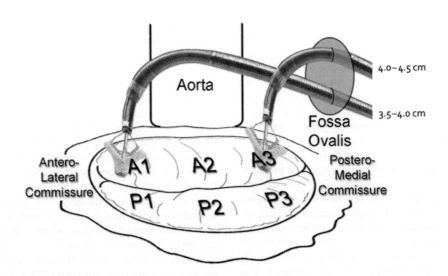

Fig. 9. The necessary height of transseptal puncture based on location of noncentral MR jet (medial vs lateral). Traditionally, higher transseptal puncture heights are needed for more medial or central MR jets, which is in contrast to more lateral jets whereby the transseptal height can be lower. As one advances the MitraClip guide catheter to the target lateral jet, height is gained.

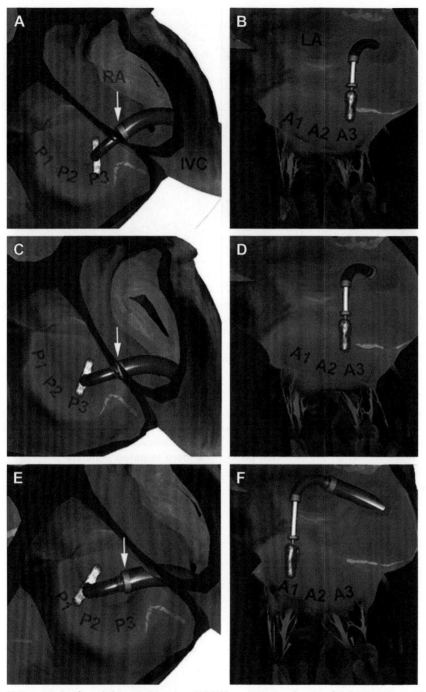

Fig. 10. (A–D) Treatment of medial regurgitant jets (A3/P3) may require the tip of the MitraClip guide (*white arrows*) to be pulled back to the interatrial septum or RA. (*E, F*) Lateral jets require the guide to be advanced more deeply into the LA, with less deflection. Because the system gains height as it crosses the LA, a relatively lower transseptal puncture site may be required. (Images generated on MitraClip Virtual Procedure Software, version 2.12.5.2, Abbott Vascular Structural Heart, Abbott Park, IL.) A1/A2/A3, segments of the anterior mitral leaflet; P1/P2/P3, scallops of the posterior mitral leaflet. (*From* Rogers JH, Low RI. Noncentral mitral regurgitation: a new niche for the MitraClip. J Am Coll Cardiol 2013;62:2379; with permission.)

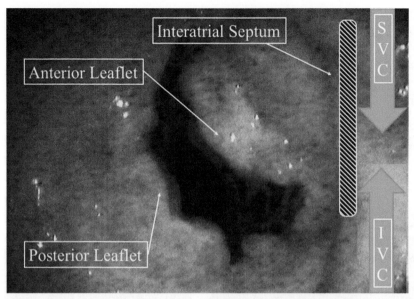

Fig. 11. Endoscopic view of the mitral valve in its normal anatomic position in the chest cavity from the posterior aspect of the LA. The mitral valve is viewed en face, and note the mitral coaptation plane is curvilinear. Additionally, the orientation of the coaptation plane and the interatrial septum (*yellow-black shaded region*) is not perpendicular. The lateral commissure is accessed easily with transseptal punctures that are more superiorly located and the medial commissure with more inferiorly located punctures. (*Courtesy of* University of Minnesota, Minneapolis, MN; with permission.)

and anchor the needle at the intended site of puncture. Alternatively, a more curved septal needle (eg, BRK-1) can be used. In cases when the needle keeps sliding off the intended puncture site, the authors find it useful to simply create a secondary bend at the location of the

RA/IVC junction (discussed later). This bend allows the needle/dilator system to exert a more perpendicular tent against the septum allowing a more targeted puncture (see Fig. 13C).

An atrial septal defect (ASD) may severely limit the ability of the operator to determine the

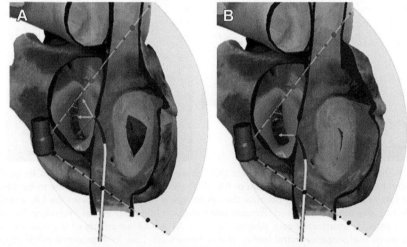

Fig. 12. En face views of the mitral and tricuspid valve from the posterior aspect of the heart with the heart in its normal anatomic position in the chest. A superior transseptal puncture (A) allows you to approach central and lateral jets (*green arrows*). However, with a superior puncture, approaching a more medial jet (*red arrow*) will require excessive flexion of the MitraClip guide catheter and may pose a greater challenge to appropriately deploy the clip. Rather, a more inferior puncture (B) allows you to directly approach a more medial jet (*green arrow*).

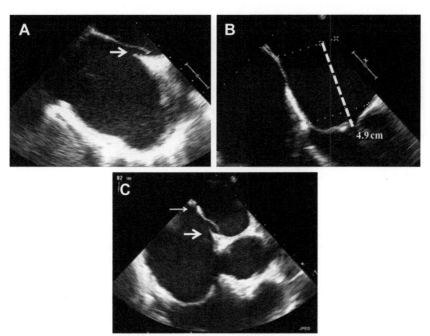

Fig. 13. The bicaval view (*A*) in this patient demonstrated a PFO (*thick arrow*). Transseptal height (*dashed line*) (*B*) at this location proved to be too high. Ultimately, a site more posterior from the PFO (*thick arrow*) was used for transseptal puncture (*thin arrow*) (*C*). From Feldman T, Franzen O, Low R, et al. Atlas of Percutaneous Edge-to-Edge Mitral Valve Repair. London: Springer; 2013; with permission.

position of a transseptal puncture and, by extension, the ability to maneuver the device. The constraints of an ASD depend on its size, location, and whether it is a single or fenestrated ASD. A very small ASD may not pose a significant problem. However, if a moderate-sized ASD is present in a suboptimal location, a transseptal puncture in the preferred location may result in a tear of the interatrial septum causing massive interatrial shunting at the conclusion of the procedure. If the ASD is in the ideal position, the MitraClip may theoretically be performed through the

defect. However, operators should be cognizant of the potential inability to properly evaluate the position of the guide, as tenting with the transseptal needle is not possible. If there is a moderate- or large-sized ASD that precludes a separate puncture location, the operator may be obligated to cross the interatrial septum through the ASD (**Fig. 14**). In some cases, this may result in issues such as insufficient height above the mitral valve. In cases such as these, MitraClip delivery may still be possible with the use of advance steering techniques.

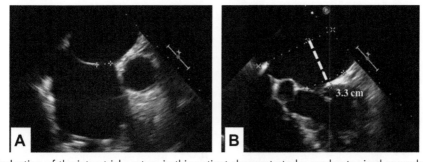

Fig. 14. Evaluation of the interatrial septum in this patient demonstrated a moderate-sized secundum ASD (*A*). Tenting at any site along the interatrial septum was not possible. Ultimately, the ASD was used to cross into the LA. The ultimate height achieved over the coaptation level was too low (*B*). However, with the use of advance steering techniques, MitraClip delivery was possible. *Dashedl line* indicates transseptal height. From Feldman T, Franzen O, Low R, et al. Atlas of Percutaneous Edge-to-Edge Mitral Valve Repair. London: Springer; 2013; with permission.

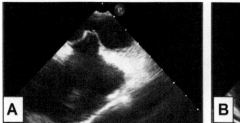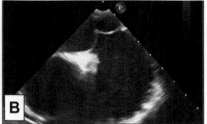

Fig. 15. X-plane view of the bicaval (*A*) and short-axis (*B*) views of a transseptal tent. Note that there is significant tenting noted with the tent approaching the posterolateral walls of the LA.

Hyperelastic Septum

Although a formal definition of a hyperelastic septum does not currently exist, this is an important entity. The authors define a hyperelastic septum as one in which greater than 1 cm of tenting persists despite appropriate forward advancement of the transseptal needle at the site of intended puncture (Fig. 15). It is yet to be determined which patient characteristics (eg, size of left/right atria, history of diastolic dysfunction, pulmonary hypertension, and so forth) predispose a patient to have a hyperelastic septum. However, the danger of a hyperelastic septum is in the so-called needle jump once the puncture has ultimately been achieved (Fig. 16). In most cases, once the intended transseptal height is engaged, gentle forward pressure is applied with the needle. In patients with significant tenting (ie, >1 cm up to several centimeters), the tent may protrude well into the LA and may encroach on vital structures (posterolateral free wall of the LA). As the puncture has yet to happen,

additional forward force may be applied by the operator creating the potential for a dangerous complication (ie, cardiac perforation) once the puncture does occur. It occurs because of the forward pressure translating into a significant needle jump, which may result in puncture of the left atrial free wall. In efforts to avert this potential complication, several different strategies can be used. One strategy would be to simply advance the accompanied mandrel or stylet, which is supplied with each BRK needle (Fig. 17). The fine tip of the mandrel will protrude through the needle tip, and this may be sufficient to create a microtear in the septum allowing the needle to puncture. Alternatively, the back end of a 0.014-in coronary guidewire can be used. If the septum can still not be punctured using these maneuvers, the use of a radiofrequency needle (eg, Baylis) may allow for more targeted puncture (Fig. 18). There remains debate in the literature and with operators regarding the use of the radiofrequency needle versus the conventional needle to achieve

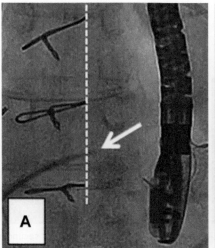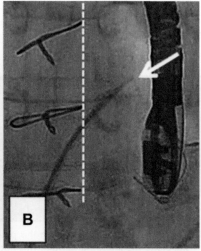

Fig. 16. Fluoroscopic image of a needle jump. (*A*) With significant tenting noted on TEE, this is a still frame from the moment just before puncture. (*B*) In the moment immediately after puncture, note the distance the system has traveled when compared with an anatomic landmark (eg, sternal wires). *Arrows* indicate needle tip.

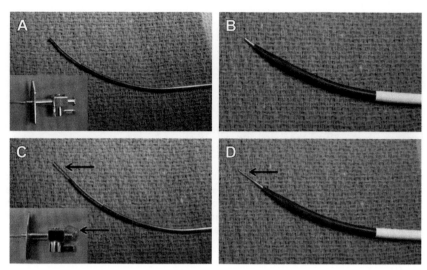

Fig. 17. Use of microwire mandrel (or stylet) to assist in transseptal puncture. In some cases the needle may slip when forward pressure is applied, and the desired location is not punctured. The wire mandrel can be used to stick the septum, thereby fixing the needle in one position and providing stabilization on needle advancement. (A) The needle alone with hub (inset). (B) The needle alone protruding from dilator. (C) The needle with wire mandrel advanced and hub detail (wire mandrel shown by arrows). (D) The needle and wire mandrel advanced out of the tip of dilator (wire mandrel shown by arrows). (From Lasala JM, Rogers JH, editors. Interventional procedures for adult structural heart disease. Philadelphia: Saunders; 2014; with permission.)

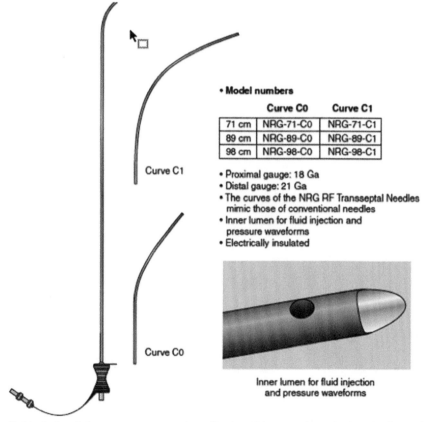

• **Model numbers**

	Curve C0	Curve C1
71 cm	NRG-71-C0	NRG-71-C1
89 cm	NRG-89-C0	NRG-89-C1
98 cm	NRG-98-C0	NRG-98-C1

• Proximal gauge: 18 Ga
• Distal gauge: 21 Ga
• The curves of the NRG RF Transseptal Needles mimic those of conventional needles
• Inner lumen for fluid injection and pressure waveforms
• Electrically insulated

Curve C1

Curve C0

Inner lumen for fluid injection and pressure waveforms

Fig. 18. Baylis Medical radiofrequency transseptal needle. As mild tenting is applied to the fossa, the needle is energized with a foot pedal. Foot pedal activation results in radiofrequency delivery to the needle tip resulting in transseptal puncture without excessive forward pressure. (Courtesy of Baylis Medical, Montreal, Quebec, Canada; with permission.)

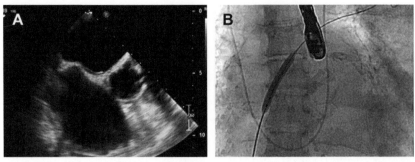

Fig. 19. Note a significant fibrotic septum in this patient with prior left-sided electrophysiologic procedures (*A*). After transseptal puncture was achieved, an 18F dilator and sheath were inserted into the right (R) femoral vein; the authors then advanced a 6 × 40-mm peripheral balloon across the septum, and atrial balloon dilatation was performed (*B*). The balloon and sheath were removed, and the guide catheter was successfully advanced across the septum and into the LA without significant resistance.

transseptal access.[8] Some operators have advocated for use of a surgical Bovie (Bovie Medical Corporation, Clearwater, FL, USA) application to the BRK needle to cauterize the way through the septum in cases of a hyperelastic septum.[9] Others prefer not to use such techniques because of the potential for coring whereby tissue fragments from the cauterized septum are still present within the hollow needle tip and may embolize to vital arterial beds.[10,11]

Fibrous Septum

Often encountered are fibrous interatrial septa whereby a thin fossa is not clearly evident (**Fig. 19**A). There are no studies reporting the patient characteristics in which a fibrous or thick interatrial septum is encountered, although anecdotally the authors have seen it in patients with prior transseptal access for cardiac electrophysiologic procedures or in patients with prior cardiac surgery with interatrial septal repair. Additionally, despite the visual appearance of a

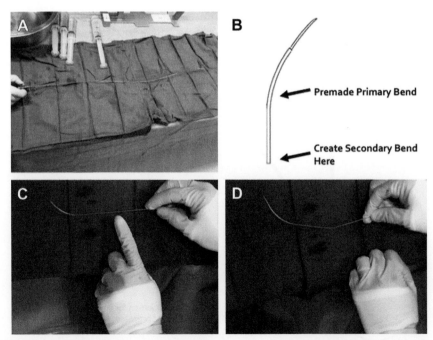

Fig. 20. (*A*) A BRK needle after it was removed from a patient with significant iliofemoral tortuosity. The tortuosity in the iliofemoral system pulls the needle away from the fossa. In cases such as these, a secondary bend is needed. (*B*) The location of the primary bend and the approximate location of where a secondary bend is created. The BRK needle immediately before (*C*) and the BRK needle immediately after (*D*) the creation of a secondary bend.

thick or fibrous septum, the transseptal puncture can be relatively easily achieved; but significant resistance can be encountered when attempting to advance the guide catheter across the septum. In cases such as these, the authors often perform balloon dilatation with a 6- to 8-mm peripheral balloon before advancing the MitraClip guide catheter (see Fig. 19B). With appropriate dilatation/stretch of the septum, the guide catheter then crosses with less resistance.

Iliofemoral Tortuosity/Enlarged Right Atrium

Encountering significant iliofemoral venous tortuosity is not uncommon in the high-risk and elderly patient population referred for transcatheter mitral valve repair. Significant tortuosity may result in inadequate tenting of the septum as the needle is pulled away from the septum from the underlying tortuosity (Fig. 20A). A similar scenario can occur in cases of left-sided venous access (when the right (R) femoral vein is occluded or compromised) or an enlarged RA. Targeted transseptal puncture is still feasible in complex scenarios such as these. Both the BRK and the Baylis needle contain a premade primary bend (see Fig. 20B). In cases that are outlined in this section, the authors particularly create a secondary bend 2 to 3 cm proximal to the primary bend (see Fig. 20C, D). This location corresponds approximately to the IVC-atrial junction. With the added bend, the tenting necessary for targeted transseptal puncture can then be achieved.

SUMMARY

Targeted transseptal puncture remains the most critical initial part of the overall MitraClip procedure. Care and attention must be implemented for patient safety in choosing the optimal puncture site. A consistent and step-by-step methodical approach is recommended. As experienced operators are targeting more complex and nontraditional pathologic conditions, the use of adjunctive tools and maneuvers (outlined in this review) are paramount to achieving successful targeted transseptal access and ultimately procedural success.

REFERENCES

1. Ross J Jr. Trans-septal left heart catheterization: a new method of left atrial puncture. Ann Surg 1959;149:395–401.
2. Ross J Jr. Transseptal left heart catheterization: a 50 year odyssey. J Am Coll Cardiol 2008;51:2107–15.
3. Roelke M, Conrad Smith AJ, Palacios IF. The technique and safety of transseptal left heart catheterization: the Massachusetts General Hospital experience with 1,279 procedures. Cathet Cardiovasc Diagn 1994;32:332–9.
4. Matsumoto T, Kar S. Latest advances in transseptal structural heart interventions: percutaneous mitral valve repair and left atrial appendage occlusion. Circ J 2014;78:1782–90.
5. Mauri L, Garg P, Massaro J, et al. The EVEREST II Trial: design and rationale for a randomized study of the Evalve MitraClip system compared with mitral valve surgery for mitral regurgitation. Am Heart J 2010;160:23–9.
6. Estevez-Loureiro R, Franzen O, Winter R, et al. Echocardiographic and clinical outcomes of central versus noncentral percutaneous edge-to-edge repair of degenerative mitral regurgitation. J Am Coll Cardiol 2013;62:2370–7.
7. Rogers JH, Low RI. Noncentral mitral regurgitation: a new niche for the MitraClip. J Am Coll Cardiol 2013;62:2378–81.
8. Hsu JC, Badhwar N, Gertenfelt EP. Randomized trial of conventional transseptal needle versus radiofrequency energy needle puncture for left atrial access (the TRAVERSE-LA Study). J Am Heart Assoc 2013;2(5):e000428.
9. Maisano F, La Canna G, Latib A, et al. Transseptal access for MitraClip procedures using surgical diathermy under echocardiographic guidance. Eurointervention 2012;8:579–86.
10. Greenstein E, Passman R, Lin AC, et al. Incidence of tissue coring during transseptal catheterization when using electrocautery and a standard transseptal needle. Circ Arrhythm Electrophysiol 2012; 5:341–4.
11. Feld G, Tiongson J, Oshodi G. Particle formation and risk of embolization during transseptal catheterization: comparison of standard transseptal needles and a new radiofrequency transseptal needle. J Interv Card Electrophysiol 2011;30:31–6.

MitraClip Therapy for Mitral Regurgitation
Primary Mitral Regurgitation

G. Athappan, MD[a], Mohammad Qasim Raza, MD[b],
Samir R. Kapadia, MD[c],*

KEYWORDS

- MitraClip • Degenerative MR • Primary MR • High risk • Mitral regurgitation

---

KEY POINTS

- Current evidence suggests MitraClip is an alternative to surgical mitral valve replacement/repair in high-risk patients with severe primary mitral regurgitation (MR).
- Surgical experience suggests that freedom from reoperation is remarkably low when annuloplasty is not performed for any reason. However, Percutaneous MitraClip therapy has different mechanical effects compared to isolated surgical alfieri stitch and is likely more durable in itself without concomitant annuloplasty.
- Percutaneous MitraClip therapy has different mechanical effects compared with the surgical Alfieri technique.
- It seems likely that the role of MitraClip in MR will expand with more novel device designs, improvements in imaging techniques, and operator experience.

BACKGROUND

Abnormalities of the mitral valve (MV) that affect closure during systole cause mitral regurgitation (MR) that can be either functional or primary. Carpentier proposed a morphologic classification[1] based on leaflet motion to describe the pathophysiologic changes that contributed to MR from either etiology (Fig. 1). Dominant leaflet pathology leading to Carpentier class II with or without class III dysfunction is the hallmark of primary MR. It is often owing to either Barlows disease (myxomatous valve disease, MV prolapse, or floppy valve) or fibroelastic deficiency. Key differences between the 2 classification systems are shown in Table 1.

The natural history of patients with chronic MR depends on the degree of regurgitation, the cause of the underlying disorder, and the degree of left ventricular (LV) dysfunction.[2–4] When severe MR is present, approximately 5% to 10% of patients per year develop significant symptoms (LV failure, pulmonary hypertension, atrial fibrillation, and stroke), clinical indications for surgery, death, or all of these.[5,6] Accordingly, the American College of Cardiology/American Heart Association and European Society of Cardiology guidelines recommend MV surgery in severe MR when symptoms supervene, or once LV dilatation (LV end-systolic diameter >40 mm) or LV dysfunction (LV ejection fraction of 30%–60%) develop.[7,8] Owing to the invasive nature of surgery and the frequent presence of comorbidities, up to 50% of patients with severe MR may not be candidates for surgery.[9] This is especially true for older patients and those with impaired LV

No funding and no disclosures for all authors.

[a] Department of Cardiovascular Medicine, Heart & Vascular Institute, Temple University Hospital, 3401 North Broad Street, Philadelphia, PA 19140, USA; [b] Department of Cardiovascular Medicine, Heart & Vascular Institute, Cleveland Clinic, 9500 Euclid Avenue, J2-3, Cleveland, OH 44195, USA; [c] Cardiac Catheterization Laboratory, Department of Cardiovascular Medicine, Heart & Vascular Institute, Cleveland Clinic, 9500 Euclid Avenue, J2-3, Cleveland, OH 44195, USA
* Corresponding author.
E-mail address: kapadis@ccf.org

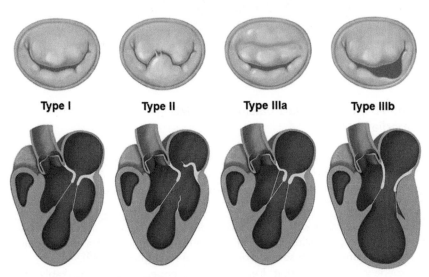

Fig. 1. Carpentier's classification of mitral regurgitation.

function. As a result, percutaneous technologies that offer the potential benefit of decreased morbidity, improved recovery time, and shorter hospital stays compared with surgery are poised to significantly alter the treatment paradigm for chronic severe MR in this group. The MitraClip is currently the only available percutaneous option that is approved by the US Food and Drug Administration (FDA) for commercial use in patients with primary MR.

MITRACLIP DEVICE

In the early 1990s, Alfieri introduced a simple and effective surgical procedure termed the "edge-to-edge repair" for the treatment of mitral regurgitation in complex lesions.[10] He and his colleagues sutured together the edges of the mitral leaflets at the site of regurgitation to treat MR. When the sutures were applied centrally, it resulted in a double orifice repair and when applied to either side it resulted in a single large orifice called a para

Table 1 Differentiation of the type of primary mitral regurgitation		
	Barlows Disease	**Fibroelastic Deficiency**
Presentation	Young adulthood	Elderly patients (>65 y)
Duration of mitral regurgitation	Long standing, with surgical referral at 40–50 y of age	Short history of mitral valve disease
Gross pathology	Chordal elongation and thickening Thick leaflets with excessive tissue Annulus is often enlarged with occasional calcification of annulus and anterior PM	Ruptured chord that is thin, sparse and frail Thin and translucent leaflets except in prolapsing segment that may be thickened Annulus may be dilated and may be calcified
Histology	Myxomatous degeneration	Thin and transparent; thickened only in the prolapsed area; "pellucid" mitral valve
Involved segments	Multiple (Prolapse or flail), bileaflet prolapse is seen in 30% of cases	Single (prolapse or flail), most common presentation is isolated P2 prolapse
Mitral valve reconstruction	Simple techniques Repair rates approach 100% Experienced general cardiac surgeon	Advanced techniques Repair rates are <100% Experienced mitral valve surgeon

commissural repair. The percutaneous edge-to-edge repair using the MitraClip system is modeled on this surgical concept and was pioneered by St Goar and colleagues.[11]

The current MitraClip device (Abbot Vascular, Menlo Park, CA) has 2 major components, a steerable guide catheter and the clip delivery system (Fig. 2).[12] The tip of the steerable guide catheter is delivered to the left atrium after a transseptal puncture. It is essential to perform the transseptal puncture relatively posterior and high in the fossa ovalis to allow adequate working space for delivery and subsequent clip placement. The ideal height for transseptal puncture from the mitral annulus is 3.5 to 4 cm. The guide catheter that is 24F proximally tapers to 22F at the point where it crosses the atrial septum. The steering knob on the back end of the guide catheter allows precise orientation and positioning of the clip. The clip delivery system with an attached clip is advanced through the guide catheter into the left atrium and then across the MV centered over the origin of the regurgitant mitral jet in an open position. Positioning of the clip over the origin of the regurgitant jet is aided by TEE. The clip is a polyester-covered cobalt chromium device with 2 arms that are opened and closed by control mechanisms on the clip delivery system. The clip has an arm span of approximately 2 cm when opened in the grasping position. The width of the clip is 4 mm. On the inner portion of the clip are 2 "grippers" that match up to each arm and helps to secure the leaflets from the atrial aspect as they are captured during closure of the clip. Leaflet tissue is secured between the arm and corresponding gripper on each side. After satisfactory reduction in MR, the clip is closed and locked to effectively achieve a double orifice repair similar to the Alfieri stitch (Figs. 3 and 4).

EXPERIENCE WITH THE MITRACLIP DEVICE FOR PRIMARY MITRAL REGURGITATION

The evidence base for FDA approval of the MitraClip system in primary MR arises from the pivotal randomized, controlled Endovascular Valve Edge-to-Edge Repair Study (EVEREST) II trial,[13,14] along with data from the EVEREST high-risk registry[15] and the Real World Expanded Multi-center Study of the MitraClip System (REALISM) registry.

THE ENDOVASCULAR VALVE EDGE-TO-EDGE REPAIR STUDY

EVEREST II was a prospective, multicenter, randomized, controlled trial designed to evaluate the safety and efficacy of percutaneous mitral repair with the MitraClip versus surgical repair or replacement for moderate to severe and severe MR in patients eligible for surgery across 37 centers in North America.[16] The primary

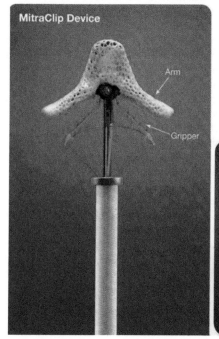

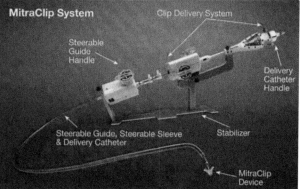

Fig. 2. Percutaneous MitraClip system. (*Courtesy of* Abbot Vascular, Menlo Park, CA; with permission.)

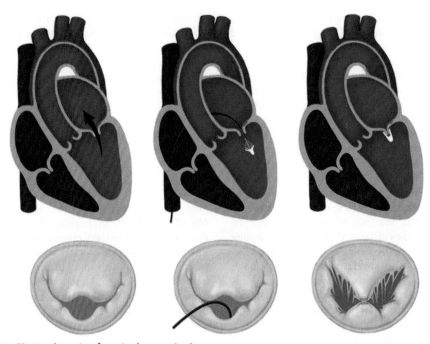

Fig. 3. MitraClip implantation for mitral regurgitation.

safety endpoint was major adverse events a composite (death, major stroke, reoperation of the MV, urgent/emergent cardiovascular surgery, myocardial infarction, renal failure, deep wound infection, ventilation for longer than 48 hours, new-onset permanent atrial fibrillation, septicemia, gastrointestinal complication requiring surgery, or transfusion of >2 U) at 30 days or hospital discharge. The primary efficacy endpoint was a composite of freedom from surgery for valve dysfunction, death, and greater than 2+ MR at 12 months. The efficacy end point between the 2 groups was compared using a margin of reduced effectiveness of 25% points in the intention-to-treat analysis and 31% points for the per protocol analysis. A total of 279 patients with severe MR were randomized in a 2:1 fashion (184 to MitraClip and 85 to surgery), 73% of whom had degenerative MR and 27% had functional MR (Box 1).

Acute procedural success defined as successful implantation of the MitraClip device with resulting MR of 2+ or less at discharge was achieved in 77% of patients (137/178) in whom it was attempted. At 30 days, the primary safety endpoint was experienced by 15% of the percutaneous group and 48% of the "control" surgical group, although it should be noted that much of this difference was accounted for by the need for transfusions of more than 2 U in the surgical group (45% in surgical arm vs 13% in MitraClip arm). With the exclusion of the need for

transfusion, the rate of major adverse events at 30 days was lower in the percutaneous repair group than in the surgery group (5% vs 10%; $P = .23$), although the difference was not significant. Notable, however, was the lack of death, major stroke, urgent or emergent surgery, or repeat MV surgery in any of the 136 patients with MitraClip who achieved APS. Freedom from death at up to 5 years of follow-up was 81.2% in the MitraClip arm and 79% in the surgical arm. An analysis of clinical effectiveness at 12 months showed the MitraClip to be "noninferior" to surgery (72.4% vs 55%; prespecified margin for noninferiority 25%), a difference that was largely driven by an increased need for surgery in the MitraClip arm (20% vs 2.2%). The reasons for surgery were no implantation of a MitraClip (17 patients), mitral regurgitation of grade greater than 2+ after device implantation before hospital discharge (n = 5), mitral regurgitation of grade greater than 2+ after attachment of a device to a single leaflet (n = 9), mitral regurgitation of grade greater than 2+ after discharge despite dual-leaflet attachment (n = 3), and symptoms (n = 3). In 7 cases, leaflet or chordae tears were noted during surgery. The overall clinical effectiveness was 39.8% in the percutaneous arm versus 53.4% in the surgical arm at 4 years of follow-up ($P = .070$). Almost all of the MitraClip–treated patients who require an additional procedure did so within the first 12 months after

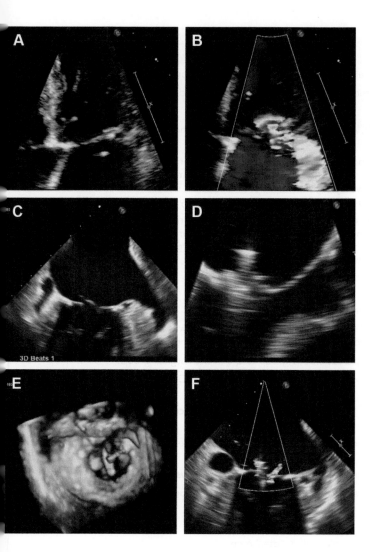

Fig. 4. Successful use of the MitraClip in primary mitral regurgitation (MR). (*A*) Two-dimensional transthoracic echocardiography showing anterior flail mitral leaflet. (*B*) Color flow Doppler showing severe eccentric MR, (*C*) Transesophageal echocardiography (TEE) of the same patient showing flail anterior leaflet. (*D*) Mitral leaflet coaptation after grasping of the valve leaflets by the MitraClip. (*E*) Positioning of the clip arms on 3-dimensional TEE. (*F*) Reduction in MR after MitraClip implantation.

initial treatment (20.4% vs 2.2%; $P = .001$). After 12 months, the rates of reoperation or additional MitraClip procedures were no different between the 2 treatment groups (24.8% vs 5.5%). At 12 months and 4 years, the proportions of patients with 3+ or 4+ MR in the percutaneous repair group were 18.8% (28/149) and 20.6% (20/97), respectively. In the surgical group the proportions of patients with 3+ or 4+ MR were 3% (2/67) and 9.1% (4/44) at 12 months and 4 years. In a subgroup analysis, MV surgery was more effective than Mitra-Clip in patients younger than 70 years of age and in those with degenerative MR.

The EVEREST II trial was criticized for selecting MR grade greater than 2+ instead of MR grade greater than 1+ as an effectiveness endpoint as MV surgery achieves MR of 1+ or less most often. Reperforming the effectiveness analyses on this revised definition as freedom from death, any surgery and MR greater than 1+ failed to meet the prespecified noninferiority margins. The MitraClip was, therefore, deemed less effective than surgery in patients suitable for surgical correction and denied approval by the FDA in patients suitable for surgical correction.[17]

INTEGRATED HIGH SURGICAL RISK PRIMARY MITRAL REGURGITATION COHORT: THE ENDOVASCULAR VALVE EDGE-TO-EDGE REPAIR STUDY II HIGH-RISK REGISTRY AND THE REAL WORLD EXPANDED MULTI-CENTER STUDY OF THE MITRACLIP SYSTEM HIGH-RISK REGISTRY

Patients enrolled in the EVEREST II high-risk study (enrollment from February 14, 2007, through January 30, 2008) and the later

Box 1
EVEREST II Randomized, controlled trial data

- The randomized, controlled trial compared conventional surgery for MR with percutaneous repair
  - 279 patients were randomized, 184 to the percutaneous arm and 95 to the surgical arm
- Procedural outcomes
  - APS achieved in 137 (76.9%). A second clip was needed during the index procedure for 38% of the patients.
  - APS was not achieved in 41 patients (23.1%) undergoing percutaneous repair. No MitraClip device was implanted in 20 patients. Of the 21 patients with MitraClip implantation and failed APS, 6 had partial leaflet detachment. Twenty-eight patients with failed APS underwent successful mitral valve surgery. APS was achieved in all patients who underwent surgery.
  - Major adverse events at 30 days were 15% in the MitraClip arm and 48% in the surgical arm. Transfusion of $\geq$2 units of blood was required by 13% in the MitraClip arm and 45% in the surgical arm. In a PP analysis, there were no deaths, stroke, MI urgent cardiovascular surgery, renal failure, deep wound infections, ventilation greater than 48 hours, or new-onset persistent A-Fib in the MitraClip group.
- Twelve-month follow-up
  - Nine patients had single leaflet detachment of the MitraClip.
  - Freedom from death, MR >2+ and surgery for MV dysfunction was seen in 55% of patients in the MitraClip group and 73% of patients in the surgical group at 12 months.
  - There were 11 deaths in the percutaneous group and 5 in the surgical group.
  - MR greater than 2+ was present in 19% of patients in the MitraClip arm and 4% of patients in the surgical arm.
  - Surgery for MR greater than 2+ was needed in 20% in the percutaneous group and 2.2% in the surgical group.
  - Reduction in left ventricular end diastolic volume was greater the surgery group (-25.3 ± 28.3 vs -40.2 ± 35.9 mL).
  - Reduction in LVEF was also greater after surgery ($-2.8 \pm 7.2\%$ vs $-6.8 \pm 10.1\%$).
  - NYHA functional class III/IV was present in 2% of patients in the percutaneous group and in 13% of those in the surgical group.
- Four-year follow-up
  - After 12 months, 1 additional single leaflet detachment.
  - There was 1 case of mitral stenosis.
  - Freedom from death, MR >2+ and surgery was 39.8% in the percutaneous arm and 53.4% in the surgical arm.
  - Freedom from death was 82.6 in the MitraClip arm and 82.2 in the surgical arm.
  - MR greater than 2+ was present in 20.6% of patients in the MitraClip arm and 9.1% of patients in the surgical arm.
  - Surgery for MR greater than 2+ was needed in 20.4% versus 2.2% at 1 year, and 24.8% versus 5.5% at 4 years. The majority of surgeries in the MitraClip group (n = 37) occurred before 12 months. Only 3 additional patients required surgery after 12 months.
  - Both groups had sustained reduction in left ventricular volumes and dimensions.
  - NYHA functional class III/IV was present in 5.7% of patients in the percutaneous group and in 6.3% of those in the surgical group.

Abbreviations: A-Fib, atrial fibrillation; APS, acute procedural success; EVEREST, Endovascular Valve Edge-to-Edge REpair Study; LVEF, left ventricular ejection fraction; MI, myocardial infarction; MR, mitral regurgitation; MV, mitral valve; NYHA, New York Heart Association; PP, per protocol.

REALISM continued access registry (enrollment began January 22, 2009, and is ongoing) with prohibitive surgical risk and primary MR were pooled to form the integrated high surgical risk primary MR cohort.[18] The EVEREST II high-risk registry was designed as an adjunctive to the EVEREST II randomized, controlled trial to evaluate the safety and efficacy of the MitraClip system in treatment of high surgical risk patients (Society of Thoracic Surgeons [STS] score >12) whereas the EVEREST II REALISM was designed to collect further safety and efficacy data beyond the enrollment period for the EVEREST II randomized, controlled trial on the "real-world" use of the MitraClip system. The REALISM study consisted of 2 arms: a high-risk group and a non–high-risk group.

Prohibitive risk for surgical repair of primary MR was identified by an STS predicted risk of 30-day mortality of at least 8% for MV replacement or if determined by the surgeon to be at high risk owing to either (1) porcelain aorta, (2) frailty (assessed by ≥2 indices), (3) hostile chest, (4) severe liver disease/cirrhosis (Model of End-stage Liver Disease score of >12), (5) severe pulmonary hypertension (systolic pulmonary artery pressure more than two-thirds systemic pressure), or (6) other unusual circumstances.

A total of 127 patients with primary MR and prohibitive surgical risk were identified by pooling the 2 registries (Box 2). Enrolled patients were elderly with a mean age of 82.4 years and with a mean prohibitive STS score of $13.2 \pm 7.3\%$. The MitraClip device was successfully implanted in 95.3% of patients (121/127). Fifty-six patients (44.1%) received a single clip, and 65 patients (51.2%) received 2 clips. Six patients (4.7%) did not have a MitraClip device implanted. The observed 30-day mortality rate was 6.3% (8 patients), substantially lower than the study population's mean STS-predicted

---

Box 2
Integrated high-risk cohort: Primary MR

- Prohibitive surgical risk patients (STS mortality ≥8%) with primary MR from the EVEREST high-risk registry and REALISM registry were pooled to form the integrated high-risk primary MR cohort.
  - Included 127 patients with MR of degenerative etiology and prohibitive surgical risk.
- Procedural outcomes
  - Successful clip implantation achieved in 95.3% of the patients (51.2% of the patients received 2 devices).
  - There were 8 deaths (6.3%), 3 strokes (2.4%), 16 major bleeding complications (12.6%), 7 major vascular complications (5.5%), 1 myocardial infarction (0.8%), 2 acute kidney injuries (1.6%), and 2 atrial septal defects (1.6%). Four patients (3.1%) required ventilation beyond 48 hours.
  - Average duration of hospital stay was 2.9 ± 3.1 days, with 88% of the patients discharged home.
  - Improvements to MR ≤2+ were observed in 62 of the 72 patients (86.1%) with baseline MR of 3+ and in 26 of the 38 (68.4%) patients with baseline 4+ MR. Improvements to MR of ≤1+ were observed in 42 of the 72 patients (58.3%) with baseline MR of 3+ and in 14 of the 38 patients (36.8%) with baseline MR of 4+.
  - NYHA functional class I or II were observed in 60 of 79 patients (75.9%) with baseline class III and in 17 of 26 patients (65.3%) with baseline class IV.
- Twelve-month follow-up
  - There were 30 deaths during the 12-month period.
  - Of 91 patients discharged with MR ≤2+, 64 patients (70.3%) sustained MR ≤2+ at 1 year, 10 (11.0%) experienced worsening MR to 3+ or 4+, and 17 (18.7%) died. Of 59 patients discharged with MR ≤1+, 21 patients (35.6%) sustained MR ≤1+ at 1 year, 20 (33.9%) experienced MR increase to 2+, 8 (13.6%) experienced worsening MR to 3+ or 4+, and 10 (16.9%) died.
  - Three patients required surgery for MV dysfunction.
  - Left-ventricular end-diastolic volume decreased significantly (125.1 ± 40.1 to 108.5 ± 37.9 mL).
  - There was a 73% decrease in heart failure hospitalizations after MitraClip therapy.

Abbreviations: EVEREST, Endovascular Valve Edge-to-Edge REpair Study; MR, mitral regurgitation; MV, mitral valve; NYHA, New York Heart Association; REALISM, Real World Expanded Multi-center Study of the MitraClip System; STS, Society of Thoracic Surgeons.

Table 2
Selection criteria in the EVEREST trials

Variable	EVEREST II	EVEREST – HRS	EVEREST-HRS-REALISM
MR severity	Grade 3+ or 4+ chronic MR	Grade 3+ or 4+ MR	Grade 3+ or 4+ MR
Clinical characteristics	Asymptomatic patients: LVEF 25%–60% or, LVESD 40–55 mm or, New-onset A-Fib or, Pulmonary hypertension OR, Symptomatic patients: LVEF ≥25% and, LVESD ≤55 mm Patients were candidates for MV repair or replacement surgery, including cardiopulmonary bypass	STS predicted risk of 30-d mortality of ≥12% Potential qualifying factors: Porcelain aorta or mobile ascending aorta atheroma or, Postmediastinal radiation or, Functional MR with LVEF <40% or, Age >75 y with LVEF <40% or, Previous median sternotomy with patent grafts or, >2 previous chest surgeries or, hepatic cirrhosis or, ≥3 of the following STS high-risk criteria: Cr >2/5 mg/dL, previous chest surgery, age >75 y, or LVEF <35%	STS predicted risk of 30-d mortality of ≥8% Potential qualifying factors: Porcelain or extensively calcified ascending aorta or, Frailty or, Hostile chest or, Severe liver disease/cirrhosis or, Severe pulmonary hypertension or, RV dysfunction with severe TR or, Chemotherapy for malignancy or, Major bleeding diathesis or, HIV/AIDS or, Severe dementia w/high risk of aspiration
Echocardiographic anatomy	The primary regurgitant jet originates from malcoaptation of the A2 and P2 scallops of the MV; if a secondary jet exists, it must be considered clinically insignificant	The primary regurgitant jet originating from malcoaptation of A2/P2 region of leaflets	All MV anatomic criteria as in previous studies

Exclusion criteria	Acute myocardial infarction in the prior 12 wk, the need for any other cardiac surgery, any endovascular or operative procedure 30 d prior, LVEF <25%, and/or end-systolic dimension >55 mm, MV orifice area <4.0 cm², if leaflet flail is present - width of the flail segment ≥15 mm or flail gap ≥10 mm, if leaflet tethering is present - coaptation depth >11 mm or vertical coaptation length <2 mm, severe mitral annular calcification, unfavorable leaflet anatomy, prior MV surgery	Acute myocardial infarction within 2 wk, LVEF <20% and/or an LV end-systolic dimension >60 mm, MV area <4.0 cm², leaflet anatomy that might preclude successful device implantation, prior history of MV leaflet surgery, echocardiographic evidence of an intracardiac mass, thrombus, or vegetation, active endocarditis	All exclusion criteria in previous studies

Abbreviations: A-Fib, atrial fibrillation; Cr, creatinine; EVEREST, Endovascular Valve Edge-to-Edge REpair Study; HIV, human immunodeficiency virus; LVEF, left ventricular ejection fraction; LVESD, left ventricular end-systolic diameter; MR, mitral regurgitation; REALISM, Real World Expanded Multi-center Study of the MitraClip System; RV, right ventricular; STS, Society of Thoracic Surgeons; TR, tricuspid regurgitation.

surgical mortality of 13.2% with surgical MV replacement. At 12 months, there were a total of 30 deaths (23.6%). Major bleeding and major vascular complications were seen in 12.6% and 5.5% of patients, respectively, at 30 days. Other safety end points are shown in **Box 2**. MR of 2+ or less at discharge was observed in 62 of the 72 patients (86.1%) with baseline MR of 3+ and in 26 of the 38 patients (68.4%) with baseline 4+ MR. MR of 1+ or less was observed in 42 of the 72 patients (58.3%) with a baseline MR of 3+ and in 14 of the 38 patients (36.8%) with a baseline MR of 4+. Ultimately, 91 patients were discharged with MR of 2+ or less. At 1 year of follow-up, 70.3% maintained MR of 2+ or less, 11% experienced worsening MR grade to 3+ or 4+, and 18.7% died. Notably, rehospitalization for heart failure was significantly decreased (73%) during the 12-month post MitraClip implantation compared with the 12 months before implantation (0.67 [95% CI, 0.54–0.83] to 0.18 [95% CI, 0.11–0.28] per patient-year). Improvements in New York Heart Association (NYHA) functional class to I or II was seen in 60 of 79 patients (75.9%) with baseline class III and in 17 of 26 patients (65.3%) with baseline class IV.

The excellent outcomes of the MitraClip in primary MR as demonstrated by the high initial success rate with a low rate of serious complications combined with sustained durability of reduction in MR leading to reduction in HF hospitalization led to FDA approval of the device for primary MR in patients with a prohibitive surgical risk.

WORLDWIDE OUTCOMES OF THE MITRACLIP IN PRIMARY MITRAL REGURGITATION

Taramasso and colleagues[19] reported outcomes on 48 consecutive high-risk patients (mean age of 78.5 ± 10.8 years and STS score of 12 ± 10%) with severe degenerative mitral regurgitation who underwent MitraClip implantation in a large-volume single center. The device was successfully implanted in 47 of 48 patients (98%) with an in-hospital mortality of 2% and no incidence of acute myocardial infarction, stroke, major vascular complication, or cardiac tamponade at 30 days. MR reduction to grade 2+ or less was observed in 43 of 47 patients (91.5%) at discharge. Actuarial survival was 89 ± 5.2% and 70.2 ± 9% at 1 and 2 years and freedom from MR of 3+ or greater was 80 ± 7% at 1 year and 76.6 ± 7% at 2 years.

In the ACCESS-EUROPE (ACCESS EU - An Observational Study of the MitraClip System in Europe),[20] a post conformité européenne (CE) approval study designed to gain information regarding the use of the MitraClip system in the European Union, 117 patients with primary MR were treated with the MitraClip device. Thirty-three of these patients were considered to be at high risk for surgical MV replacement with a logistic Euroscore of 33.1 ± 11.5. Twenty-nine patients underwent successful device implantation with an in-hospital mortality of 9.1% (3/33) and any adverse events in 27.3% (9/33). MR reduction to grade less than 1+ at discharge was achieved in 48.3% (14/29). Over a period of 12 months, observed mortality was 24.2% (8/33) and freedom from MR greater than grade 2+ and NYHA functional class I or II was seen in 80% and 57.1% of patients, respectively.

INDICATIONS AND PATIENT SELECTION

The MitraClip Clip has been approved by the FDA for percutaneous reduction of significant symptomatic degenerative MR of 3+ or greater in patients who have been determined by a cardiac surgeon to be too high risk for open MV surgery. The determination of high risk is based on the EVEREST high-risk criteria[15] (**Table 2**). In addition to determination of high risk, suitability for the MitraClip procedure requires echocardiographic anatomic assessment of the MV. In the EVEREST trails[4,21] and continued access registry the implantation of the MitraClip was limited to patients with predominantly central (A2/P2) MR, mitral orifice area of greater than 4 cm^2, flail gap of less than 10 mm, and flail width of less than 15 mm. Calcification of the valve leaflets in the grasping area was considered a contraindication to clipping owing to the potential risk of clip embolization. Additionally, mitral annular calcification if severe was excluded from the EVEREST II trial to maximize the probability of valve repair in patients randomized to the surgical arm.

There is, however, accumulating evidence to support the use of the MitraClip in degenerative MR with more complex morphologies. Estévez-Loureiro and colleagues[22] compared the outcomes of Mitraclip implantation in central versus noncentral MR from 3 high-volume centers in Europe. Procedural success was the same in both groups (95.5% central vs 96.7% noncentral), as were postprocedural adverse events: partial clip detachment (2.0% central vs 3.3% noncentral) and death (5.4% central vs 13.0% noncentral). Postprocedural MR and NYHA functional class at 1 month were also similar in both groups (MR ≤2, 96.0% central vs 96.6% noncentral; and NYHA functional class ≤II, 81.6% central vs 90.0% noncentral). Franzen and colleagues[23] showed excellent results with Mitraclip implantation despite a MV orifice area of less than 4 cm^2, flail width of greater than 15 mm, flail gap greater than 10 mm, LV ejection fraction less than 20%, and coaptation length of less than 2 mm. Similarly, in the Hamburg registry Lubos and colleagues[24] showed that a MV orifice area of less than 4 cm^2 was not a contraindication to MitraClip implantation. They identified effective regurgitant orifice area of greater than 70.8 mm^2, MV orifice area of 3 cm^2 or less and a transmitral peak gradient of 4 mm Hg or greater to predict procedural failure with MitraClip implantation. In our experience, severe mitral annular calcification also increases the risk of procedural failure and subsequent mitral stenosis if aggressively clipped (>1 clip).

SUMMARY

Percutaneous MV repair is a rapidly evolving field. The most advanced technique with the greatest safety and efficacy, to date, is the edge-to-edge MitraClip repair system. Current evidence suggests that the MitraClip is a valuable alternative to surgical MV replacement/repair in select high-risk or prohibitive surgical risk patients with severe primary MR. Data from the EVEREST II trial suggest that the MitraClip is durable for up to 4 years. Data on long-term efficacy beyond 4 years are, however, scarce. Surgical experience suggests that freedom from reoperation is remarkably low when annuloplasty is not performed for any reason. In degenerative MR, the overall long-term results of the surgical edge-to-edge technique without annuloplasty were found to be unsatisfactory by Alfieri and colleagues.[25] Despite the analogy, percutaneous MitraClip therapy has different mechanical effects compared with the surgical Alfieri technique. Percutaneous clipping exerts greater forces on the MV apparatus as compared with the operative technique leading to a decrease in annular area and diameter comparable with surgical or percutaneous annuloplasty.[26] There is an immediate decrease in annular measurements independent of late ventricular reverse remodeling. Efficacy of the Mitraclip is, therefore, likely to be durable unlike its surgical counterpart at longer follow-up. Looking forward, it does seem likely that the role of MitraClip in the treatment of MR will expand further with more novel device designs and improvements in imaging techniques and operator experience.

REFERENCES

1. Carpentier A. Cardiac valve surgery–the "French correction". J Thorac Cardiovasc Surg 1983;86: 323–37.
2. Enriquez-Sarano M, Avierinos JF, Messika-Zeitoun D, et al. Quantitative determinants of the outcome of asymptomatic mitral regurgitation. N Engl J Med 2005;352:875–83.
3. Gillinov AM, Blackstone EH, Rajeswaran J, et al. Ischemic versus degenerative mitral regurgitation: does etiology affect survival? Ann Thorac Surg 2005;80:811–9 [discussion: 809].
4. Ling LH, Enriquez-Sarano M, Seward JB, et al. Clinical outcome of mitral regurgitation due to flail leaflet. N Engl J Med 1996;335:1417–23.
5. Rosenhek R, Rader F, Klaar U, et al. Outcome of watchful waiting in asymptomatic severe mitral regurgitation. Circulation 2006;113:2238–44.
6. Rosen SE, Borer JS, Hochreiter C, et al. Natural history of the asymptomatic/minimally symptomatic patient with severe mitral regurgitation secondary to mitral valve prolapse and normal right and left ventricular performance. Am J Cardiol 1994;74: 374–80.
7. Nishimura RA, Otto CM, Bonow RO, et al. 2014 AHA/ACC guideline for the management of patients with valvular heart disease: a report of the American College of Cardiology/American Heart Association Task Force on Practice Guidelines. J Am Coll Cardiol 2014;63:e57–185.
8. Vahanian A, Alfieri O, Andreotti F, et al. Guidelines on the management of valvular heart disease (version 2012). Eur Heart J 2012;33:2451–96.
9. Mirabel M, Iung B, Baron G, et al. What are the characteristics of patients with severe, symptomatic, mitral regurgitation who are denied surgery? Eur Heart J 2007;28:1358–65.
10. Alfieri O, Maisano F, De Bonis M, et al. The double-orifice technique in mitral valve repair: a simple solution for complex problems. J Thorac Cardiovasc Surg 2001;122:674–81.
11. St Goar FG, Fann JI, Komtebedde J, et al. Endovascular edge-to-edge mitral valve repair: short-term results in a porcine model. Circulation 2003;108: 1990–3.
12. Young A, Feldman T. Percutaneous mitral valve repair. Curr Cardiol Rep 2014;16:443.
13. Feldman T, Foster E, Glower DD, et al. Percutaneous repair or surgery for mitral regurgitation. N Engl J Med 2011;364:1395–406.
14. Mauri L, Foster E, Glower DD, et al. 4-year results of a randomized controlled trial of percutaneous repair versus surgery for mitral regurgitation. J Am Coll Cardiol 2013;62:317–28.
15. Whitlow PL, Feldman T, Pedersen WR, et al. Acute and 12-month results with catheter-based mitral

valve leaflet repair: the EVEREST II (endovascular valve edge-to-edge repair) high risk study. J Am Coll Cardiol 2012;59:130–9.

16. Mauri L, Garg P, Massaro JM, et al. The EVEREST II Trial: design and rationale for a randomized study of the evalve MitraClip system compared with mitral valve surgery for mitral regurgitation. Am Heart J 2010;160:23–9.

17. Minha S, Torguson R, Waksman R. Overview of the 2013 Food and Drug Administration circulatory system devices panel meeting on the MitraClip delivery system. Circulation 2013;128:864–8.

18. Lim DS, Reynolds MR, Feldman T, et al. Improved functional status and quality of life in prohibitive surgical risk patients with degenerative mitral regurgitation after transcatheter mitral valve repair. J Am Coll Cardiol 2014;64:182–92.

19. Taramasso M, Maisano F, Denti P, et al. Percutaneous edge-to-edge repair in high-risk and elderly patients with degenerative mitral regurgitation: midterm outcomes in a single-center experience. J Thorac Cardiovasc Surg 2014;148:2743–50.

20. Reichenspurner H, Schillinger W, Baldus S, et al. Clinical outcomes through 12 months in patients with degenerative mitral regurgitation treated with the MitraClip(r) device in the ACCESS-Europe Phase I trial. Eur J Cardiothorac Surg 2013;44:e280–8.

21. Feldman T, Kar S, Rinaldi M, et al. Percutaneous mitral repair with the MitraClip system: Safety and midterm durability in the initial EVEREST (Endovascular Valve Edge-to-edge Repair Study) cohort. J Am Coll Cardiol 2009;54:686–94.

22. Estévez-Loureiro R, Franzen O, Winter R, et al. Echocardiographic and clinical outcomes of central versus noncentral percutaneous edge-to-edge repair of degenerative mitral regurgitation. J Am Coll Cardiol 2013;62:2370–7.

23. Franzen O, Baldus S, Rudolph V, et al. Acute outcomes of MitraClip therapy for mitral regurgitation in high-surgical-risk patients: emphasis on adverse valve morphology and severe left ventricular dysfunction. Eur Heart J 2010;31:1373–81.

24. Lubos E, Schluter M, Vettorazzi E, et al. MitraClip therapy in surgical high-risk patients: Identification of echocardiographic variables affecting acute procedural outcome. JACC Cardiovasc Interv 2014;7: 394–402.

25. De Bonis M, Lapenna E, Maisano F, et al. Long-term results (</=18 years) of the edge-to-edge mitral valve repair without annuloplasty in degenerative mitral regurgitation: implications for the percutaneous approach. Circulation 2014;130: S19–24.

26. Schmidt FP, von Bardeleben RS, Nikolai P, et al. Immediate effect of the MitraClip procedure on mitral ring geometry in primary and secondary mitral regurgitation. Eur Heart J Cardiovasc Imaging 2013;14:851–7.

MitraClip Therapy for Mitral Regurgitation
Secondary Mitral Regurgitation

Ted Feldman, MD, FESC, MSCAI*, Arjun Mehta, MD,
Mayra Guerrero, MD, FSCAI, Justin P. Levisay, MD, FSCAI,
Michael H. Salinger, MD, FSCAI

KEYWORDS

- MitraClip • Mitral regurgitation • COAPT • Functional mitral regurgitation

---

KEY POINTS

- Both conventional surgery and medical therapy have limited efficacy for patients with functional MR, and surgery has limited application especially in older, high risk patients.
- MitraClip has demonstrated improvements in symptoms, favorable left ventricular remodeling, and reduced heart failure hospitalizations in high risk patients with severe MR in prospective registries.
- The randomized COAPT Trial will compare MitraClip with medical therapy to better define the role of this interventional approach.

Therapy for mitral regurgitation (MR) has been synonymous with mitral valve surgery for several decades. Surgical approaches for primary or degenerative MR have been highly successful. Mitral repair for degenerative MR has been associated with excellent acute and long-term results, with durable repair in a majority of patients. In contrast, surgical correction of secondary MR owing to ischemic or dilated cardiomyopathy has not proven to be as successful (Table 1), and has limited recommended indications in the current valve therapy guidelines (Table 2).[1]

Secondary or functional MR (FMR) represents, as its name suggests, is a secondary disease, related to dilatation or geometric distortion of the left ventricular (LV) chamber. Thus, as a disease of the left ventricle, mitral valve repair or even replacement for secondary MR has had less salutary results than surgery for degenerative MR.

The benefits of decreasing the severity of MR in secondary MR using surgical annuloplasty or valve replacement have been limited.[2] There has not been any clear benefit in mortality associated with reduction of MR in this population. Several studies have showed improvements in symptoms or surrogate measures of benefit, such as favorable LV remodeling, but improvements in these nonclinical endpoints have not translated into benefits in mortality, and in fact for the population of patients with ischemic MR, survival has been poor.

Over the last several years, percutaneous options for therapy for FMR have emerged.[3] The MitraClip device has by far the greatest use in clinical practice. MitraClip is the only percutaneous leaflet therapy available in this category (Fig. 1). Other device approaches including indirect and direct annuloplasty and transcatheter mitral valve replacement have been or are being developed.

The MitraClip device was modeled based on surgical double orifice or edge-to-edge mitral repair.[4] This operative approach was developed by Ottavio Alfieri in the early 1990s.[5] Alfieri used

---

NorthShore University HealthSystem, Evanston, IL, USA
* Corresponding author. Cardiology Division, Evanston Hospital, Walgreen Building 3rd Floor, 2650 Ridge Avenue, Evanston, IL 60201.
E-mail address: tfeldman@tfeldman.org

Intervent Cardiol Clin 5 (2016) 83–91
http://dx.doi.org/10.1016/j.iccl.2015.08.007
2211-7458/16/$ – see front matter © 2016 Elsevier Inc. All rights reserved.

Table 1
Therapy options for mitral regurgitation

Surgical risk	Degenerative	Functional
Low	Surgical mitral repair	?
High	Commercial MitraClip	Global practice COAPT

Degenerative MR and low surgical risk candidates are best treated with surgery. MitraClip now offers an option for degenerative etiology patients with high surgical risk. There remains uncertainty regarding surgical treatment for functional MR. High surgical risk patients with functional MR are treated with MitraClip in international practice.

simple sutures to approximate the free edges of the mitral leaflets in patients with mitral prolapse. The methodology of this repair was to obliterate the prolapse segment and reestablish leaflet approximation. Thus, the initial intended use of the MitraClip device was for patients with degenerative MR. It was recognized early during the phase I trial experience that percutaneous MitraClip therapy could be applied to patients with FMR. It is important to remember that the original MitraClip trials were designed when the 1998 valve guidelines were current. The indications for surgical mitral valve intervention at the time did not distinguish between degenerative and functional.

The sequence of trial and registry experience with the MitraClip device has defined the current landscape for use of this therapy both in global practice and in ongoing trials. Ultimately, the MitraClip has come to be used primarily for FMR outside of the United States. In the United States, the MitraClip is commercially approved by the US Food and Drug Administration (FDA) for use in patients with degenerative MR, but remains investigational for use in patients with FMR. The journey to reach this point in current use of the therapy began with the Endovascular Valve Edge-to-Edge Repair (EVEREST) II randomized trial.

The EVEREST II trial was the key step in defining the initial role of the MitraClip device.[6] It was a randomized trial comparing percutaneous repair with conventional surgery for MR. It was designed with the inclusion criteria based on the 1998 valve guidelines. Patients were included if they had moderate to severe or severe MR with symptoms, or in the absence of symptoms had evidence of decreased LV ejection fraction or increased LV end-systolic dimensions. The MR had to originate from malcoaptation of the central portion of the line of coaptation. All of the echocardiographic findings were assessed by a core laboratory. Patients had to be candidates for mitral valve surgery, including cardiopulmonary bypass, and transseptal puncture had to be feasible. The main exclusion criteria were a LV ejection fraction of less than 25%, LV end-systolic dimension of greater than 55 mm, renal insufficiency, or history of endocarditis or rheumatic heart disease. As a result of these inclusion and exclusion criteria, a population composed of predominantly degenerative MR patients (73%) was selected. Despite the predominance of degenerative disease, one-quarter of the patients ultimately included in the trial had FMR. The main findings of the randomized comparison after 1 year, at the time of the primary endpoint assessment, were that surgery is more effective at reducing MR severity and percutaneous repair with the MitraClip device is safer. Importantly, both therapies had similar effectiveness in improving quality-of-life measures and symptoms and both were effective in leading to improved LV chamber dimensions and volumes through favorable remodeling. Subgroup analysis in this trial showed outcomes closest to those of surgery for patients with older age, worse ventricular function, and, most important, a functional etiology for MR.

Table 2
Summary of valve guideline recommendations for chronic severe secondary MR

Recommendation	Class	Level of Evidence
MV surgery is reasonable for patients with chronic severe secondary MR (stages C and D) who are undergoing coronary artery bypass grafting or aortic valve replacement	IIa	C
MV surgery may be considered for severely symptomatic patients (NYHA class III/IV) with chronic severe secondary MR (stage D)	IIb	B
MV repair may be considered for patients with chronic moderate secondary MR (stage B) who are undergoing other cardiac surgery	IIb	C

Abbreviations: MR, mitral regurgitation; MV, mitral valve; NYHA, New York Heart Association.

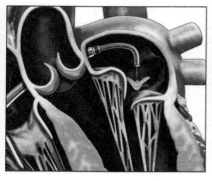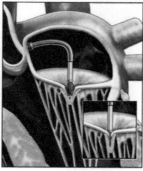

Fig. 1. To introduce the clip, the clip delivery system is advanced through the guide into the left atrium (*left*). Under echocardiographic and fluoroscopic guidance, the clip is aligned perpendicular to the valve plane, with the clip arms perpendicular to the line of coaptation. It is then advanced into the left ventricle and then slowly retracted to grasp the leaflets (*right*). The clip is closed (*right, inset*), and if reduction of mitral regurgitation is satisfactory, it is released. (*From* Feldman T, Young A. Percutaneous approaches to valve repair for mitral regurgitation. J Am Coll Cardiol 2014;63:2059; with permission.)

During the course of enrollment for the randomized trial, it was recognized that many patients were being referred for evaluation who were not candidates for surgery and thus not eligible for the trial, but had mitral anatomy ideal for MitraClip therapy and were clinically well-suited for the percutaneous MitraClip therapy (Figs. 2–4). Most of these patients were not candidates for surgery owing to advanced age and multiple comorbidities. They represented a group for whom there were no options for effective therapy. A registry was created to allow the use of MitraClip in this group.[7] This high-risk registry was composed of the types of patients who are now predominantly the MitraClip candidate population. Many lessons were learned from the high-risk registry. The 1-year outcomes have been reported. In these studies, 351 patients were included.[8] Patients were elderly with a mean age of 76 years. In contrast with the EVEREST II population, 70% had FMR. The MitraClip device reduced MR severity to 2+ or

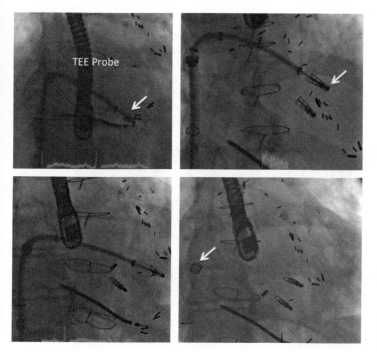

Fig. 2. Fluoroscopic images from a MitraClip procedure in a Cardiovascular Outcomes Assessment of the MitraClip Percutaneous Therapy for Heart Failure Patients with Functional Mitral Regurgitation (COAPT) patient. The patient is a 72-year-old man with severe mitral regurgitation, elevated brain natriuretic peptide, multiple heart failure hospitalizations, and additional risks of prior coronary bypass surgery, carotid endarterectomy, and chronic kidney disease. The left ventricular ejection fraction is 45%. The Society of Thoracic Surgeons risk score for mitral valve replacement is 10.9%. The upper left panel shows the placement of a MitraClip with transesophageal echo guidance (TEE). The white arrow shows the MitraClip device still attached to the delivery system. The upper panel shows placement of the second clip, noted by the arrow. This second clip is being passed lateral to the first, in a closed configuration. Lower left shows the second clip opened in the left ventricle before being pulled back to grasp the mitral leaflets. The lower right panel shows both clips after final release. The distal marker at the tip of the guide catheter is seen at the left side of the picture (*arrow*).

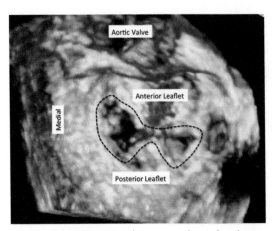

Fig. 3. Three-dimensional transesophageal echocardiographic image obtained from the left atrial. This is the so-called surgeons review. The aortic valve is at the top of the picture. The dotted black line encircles the double orifice created by placement of the MitraClips.

less in 86% of patients. The safety of the device and procedure that had been noted in prior studies were maintained in this high-risk population. Major adverse events at 30 days included death in 4.8%, myocardial infarction in 1.1%, and stroke in 2.6%. These outcomes are notable in this highly complex patient group with a predicted hospital mortality of 12% to 18%. At 12 months, MR was 2+ or less in 84%. At the 1-year time point, LV end-diastolic volume improved significantly. Symptoms were also improved, with a New York Heart Association (NYHA) functional class improved from 82% in class III/IV at baseline to 83% in class I/II at 12 months. Quality-of-life measures improved

as well. One of the most important findings from this experience was a decrease in the annual hospitalization rate for heart failure. The proportion of patients hospitalized for heart failure was reduced from 42% in the year before the procedure to 19.8% in the year after the procedure (P<.0001). Kaplan–Meier survival estimate at 12 months was 77.2%. Thus, the MitraClip device significantly reduced MR, improved clinical symptoms, and decreased LV dimensions at 12 months in this high surgical risk cohort.

The MitraClip device received CE Mark approval in 2008. Since then, more than 20,000 procedures have been done internationally. The predominant patient population are patients at high risk for surgery, often referred by cardiac surgeons, with functional or secondary MR. Several broad conclusions can be drawn from an aggregate of reports from this global practice experience. The MitraClip procedure is safe, even in this critically ill patient group. It can be performed with a procedural success rate approaching 100%. More than 85% of patients are discharged within a few days and directly to home rather than to any kind of rehabilitation facility. Clinical outcomes are excellent with the majority of patients in functional class I or II at 1 year after therapy. These results have been achieved in a wide range of mitral leaflet anatomic subsets, and patient compromised LV function.

The low mortality of MitraClip interventions is illustrated in a recently published metaanalysis that identified 21 studies in high-risk patients, representing this international experience, using the MitraClip in 3198 patients and mitral surgery in 53,265, with a mean age of 74 years.[9]

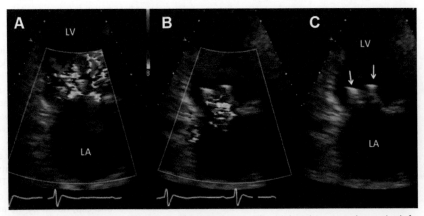

Fig. 4. Transthoracic echocardiogram obtained before discharge. This 4-chamber view shows the left ventricle (LV) at the top of the picture, and the left atrium (LA) at the bottom of the picture. (A) Double jets of diastolic inflow into the left ventricle created by the double orifice. (B) Mild mitral regurgitation into the left atrium. (C) Echocardiographic appearance of the 2 MitraClips (arrows).

Technical success was achieved in 96% of patients undergoing MitraClip and 98% in the surgery group. The pooled event rate for mortality was 3.2% and stroke 1.1% at 30 days. From 1 month to 1 year, the pooled event rate for mortality was 13.0%, stroke 1.6%, and repeat surgery 1.3%, with the majority of patients in the mild/moderate MR grade and NYHA class II or lower after MitraClip. The 30-day event rates for mortality and stroke were 16.8% and 4.5% after mitral surgery. Based on high-risk data predominantly from the Society of Thoracic Surgeons database, patients with severe MR can be treated effectively with MitraClip or surgery. The MitraClip can be implanted safely in high-risk patients with a relatively low 30-day mortality of only 3.2% in a group with a predicted mortality of greater than 15%.

A report from the German TRAnscatheter Mitral valve Interventions (TRAMI) Registry shows the high likelihood of discharge to home after MitraClip procedures in elderly, high-risk patients.[10] These investigators reported outcomes in more than 1000 patients, one-half of whom were over age 75 years with a Society of Thoracic Surgeons risk of 11.5%. The combined intrahospital rate of death, myocardial infarction, and stroke was only 3.4%. Regular discharge to home was possible in more than 80% of this risk group.

Franzen and associates[11] were among the first to demonstrate that the MitraClip could be used in patients with severely depressed LV function. MitraClip therapy was performed in 51 consecutive patients with a mean age of 73 years with symptomatic functional (69%) or organic MR (31%). The LV ejection fraction was 36 ± 17%. MitraClip implantation was successful in 96%. Procedure-related reduction in MR severity was 1 grade in 31%, 2 grades in 47%, and 3 grades in 18%. At discharge, 90% showed clinical improvement in NYHA class. There were no procedure-related major adverse events and no in-hospital mortality. Mitral valve repair using the MitraClip system was shown to be feasible in patients at high surgical risk, primarily determined by an adverse mitral valve morphology and/or severe LV dysfunction.

An important finding among patients with poor LV function and severe MR was that cardiac resynchronization therapy (CRT) nonresponders might have some benefit from MitraClip. Fifty-one severely symptomatic CRT nonresponders with significant FMR grade 2 or greater underwent MitraClip treatment.[12] MitraClip treatment was feasible in all patients. There were 2 periprocedural deaths. Median follow-up was 14 months. NYHA functional class improved acutely at discharge in 73% and continued to improve progressively during follow-up. The proportion of patients with significant residual FMR grade of 2 or greater progressively decreased during follow-up. Reverse LV remodeling and improved LV ejection fraction were detected at 6 months, with further improvement at 12 months. The overall 30-day mortality was 4.2%. Overall mortality during follow-up was 19.9 per 100 person-years. Nonsurvivors had more compromised clinical baseline conditions, longer QRS duration, and a more dilated heart. FMR treatment with the MitraClip in CRT nonresponders was feasible, safe, and demonstrated improved functional class, increased LV ejection fraction, and reduced ventricular volumes in about 70% of these study patients. Similar finding were reported by a German group.[13] This study evaluated 42 patients with CRT and MR 3+ of greater who received the MitraClip device. Thirty-six of them had CRT prior the MitraClip procedure (CRT nonresponders) and 6 had a CRT device implanted after the MitraClip device. Implantation of the MtiraClip device reduced MR to 2+ or less in 95%. In the median follow-up interval of 11.3 months, 8 patients died and 2 patients received an LV assist device. An additional patient had mitral replacement surgery 4 months after MitraClip implantation for increased MR. MitraClip implantation led to an improvement of N-terminal of the prohormone brain natriuretic peptide level, tricuspid regurgitation pressure gradient and LVEDV. After 1 year, all-cause mortality was 14%, and 2-year all-cause mortality was 25%. Patients with an N-terminal of the prohormone brain natriuretic peptide level greater than 7000 pg/mL at the time of MitraClip implantation had a significantly poorer outcome compared with patients of 7000 pg/mL or less (P = .035). Similarly, patients with reduced right ventricular function (tricuspid annular plane systolic excursion ≤15 mm) or a higher pulmonary systolic pressure (tricuspid regurgitation peak gradient >35 mm Hg) had a significant inferior outcome compared with the rest of the cohort.

A recent report demonstrates clinical benefits out to 1 year even for heart failure patients with severely depressed LV function, and also helps to define the limits of MitraClip use.[14] Thirty-four patients with an LV ejection fraction of 25% and severe MR treated with MitraClip were analyzed. MR could be successfully reduced to grade 2+ or less in 88%. Long-term follow-up up to 5 years revealed a steep decline of the survival curve reaching 50% at only

8 months after MitraClip. In contrast, estimated survival of the remaining patients showed a favorable long-term outcome. Patients who died during the first year presented with higher right ventricular pressures as estimated by systolic tricuspid regurgitant velocities (44.5 vs 35.2 mm Hg; $P<.035$) and worse right ventricular function ($P<.014$) before the procedure. One-year mortality of patients with pulmonary hypertension and depressed right ventricular function was very high (77%) compared with the remaining patients (mortality rate of 0%; $P<.0001$). Although the MitraClip leads to a successful reduction of MR in patients with an LV ejection fraction 25%, the 1-year mortality in this cohort was very high. However, a subgroup of patients showed a favorable long-term outcome after MitraClip therapy. The authors concluded that the right ventricular parameters of sustained right ventricular function and absence of pulmonary hypertension, easily assessed with echocardiography, might be used to identify the subgroup of patients with poor LV function who could be anticipated to respond favorably to MitraClip and could encourage MitraClip therapy in these patients.

Another important lesson from the global experience with MitraClip has been to extend the range of mitral leaflet anatomy that can be treated. The original EVEREST II trial had anatomic selection criteria based on the understanding of the device at that early time period in its use. A multicenter analysis sought to compare clinical outcomes in high-risk patients with moderate-to-severe to severe MR treated with the MitraClip device, stratified by whether they met the original EVEREST II echocardiographic anatomic criteria (EVEREST-ON) or not (EVEREST-OFF).[15] Acute device success was defined as residual MR 2+ or greater after clip implantation. The primary safety endpoint was the incidence of MAEs at 30 days, defined as the composite of death, myocardial infarction, reoperation for failed MitraClip implantation, nonelective cardiovascular surgery for adverse events, stroke, renal failure, deep wound infection, mechanical ventilation for longer than 48 hours, gastrointestinal complication requiring surgery, new onset of permanent atrial fibrillation, septicemia, and transfusion of 2 U of blood. The primary efficacy endpoint was freedom from death, surgery for MV dysfunction, or grade 3+ or greater MR at the 12-month follow-up after clip implantation. Seventy-eight patients were included in EVEREST-OFF and 93 patients in EVEREST-ON groups. Acute procedural success was comparable between the 2 groups

(EVEREST-OFF 97.8% vs EVEREST-ON 100.0%; $P=.294$). There was no difference in the primary safety endpoint with 2 patients (2.6%) and 6 (6.5%) in the EVEREST-OFF and EVEREST-ON groups, respectively ($P=.204$) experiencing safety events. Kaplan–Meier freedom from death, surgery for MV dysfunction, or grade 3+ or greater MR at 12 months (primary efficacy endpoint) was demonstrated in 71.4% and 76.2%, respectively, in the EVEREST-OFF and EVEREST-ON groups (log-rank $P=.378$). The components of the primary efficacy endpoint were also similar between the 2 groups. The authors concluded that MitraClip implantation in patients with expanded baseline echocardiographic features, compared with the control group, was associated with similar rates of safety and efficacy through 12-month follow-up.

Although our accumulated experience with the MitraClip seems to define a primary application for high-risk patients with FMR, FDA approval for the MitraClip in the United States is for higher risk patients with degenerative MR. This approval is based on recognition that there has not been a clear comparison of outcomes of MitraClip therapy with best medical therapy for FMR, and although surgery is clearly the preferred therapy for degenerative MR, there remains a population with degenerative MR that have risks that preclude surgery. The MitraClip thus answers an important and unmet need in this group.

The FDA approval is based on an analysis of a subgroup of the high-risk registry population.[16] A high-risk degenerative MR group of 127 patients were retrospectively identified as meeting the definition of prohibitive risk.[17] Patients were elderly with a mean age older than 82 years, severely symptomatic with 87% NYHA class III/IV, and at prohibitive surgical risk based on a Society of Thoracic Surgeons score of 13.2 ± 17.3%. The MitraClip procedure was successfully performed in more than 95% of these patients. Duration of hospital stay was fewer than 3 days. Major adverse events at 30 days included death in 6.3%, myocardial infarction in 0.8%, and stroke in 2.4%. Through 1 year, there were a total of 30 deaths (23.6%). At 1 year, the majority of surviving patients (82.9%) remained with MR 2+ or less, and 86.9% were in NYHA functional class I or II. The LV end-diastolic volume decreased significantly. Quality-of-life scores improved. Hospitalizations for heart failure were decreased among patients whose MR was reduced. Thus, in prohibitive surgical risk patients, the MitraClip is associated with safety and good clinical outcomes, including decreases in rehospitalization, functional improvements, and favorable ventricular remodeling, at 1 year.

Despite the wide use of the MitraClip in global practice for the FMR population, best therapy for patients with FMR is not defined clearly. FMR, particularly of ischemic etiology, has never had effective therapy options (see Table 1). Historically, medical therapy has had no impact. CRT has been the only successful intervention in this group. CRT is limited to a relatively small proportion of the whole population with FMR. Many patients are nonresponders to CRT. Surgery to repair or replace the mitral

---

Box 1
COAPT trial inclusion and exclusion criteria

Key inclusion criteria

- Symptomatic functional MR ($\geq$3+) of either ischemic or nonischemic etiology
- Adequately treated per applicable standards in the judgment of the HF specialist investigator
- Not an appropriate candidate for open mitral valve surgery in the judgment of the local site heart team (cardiothoracic surgeon and HF specialist investigators)
- NYHA functional class II, III, or ambulatory IV
- At least 1 hospitalization for heart failure in the 12 months before subject registration and/or a corrected BNP $\geq$300 pg/mL or corrected N-terminal of the prohormone brain natriuretic peptide $\geq$1500 pg/mL measured within 90 days before subject registration
- Primary regurgitant jet is noncommissural, and per the MitraClip implanting investigator can be successfully treated by the MitraClip (and if secondary jet exists, is clinically insignificant)
- Transseptal catheterization and femoral vein access is feasible
- Left ventricular ejection fraction is $\geq$20% and $\leq$50%
- Left ventricular end systolic dimension is $\leq$70 mm

Key exclusion criteria

- CABG within prior 30 days
- Tricuspid and/or aortic valve disease requiring surgery
- Untreated clinically significant CAD requiring revascularization
- Cerebrovascular accident within 30 days before subject registration, modified Rankin scale $\geq$4 disability or severe symptomatic carotid stenosis (>70% by ultrasound)
- ACC/AHA Stage D heart failure
- Physical evidence of right-sided congestive heart failure with echo evidence of moderate or severe RV dysfunction
- PCI or carotid surgery within prior 30 days
- Implant of any CRT or CRT-D within the last 30 days before subject registration
- Mitral valve orifice area <4.0 cm^2, or leaflet anatomy that might preclude MitraClip implantation
- Life expectancy <12 months owing to noncardiac conditions
- Hemodynamic instability requiring inotropic support or other hemodynamic support device
- Need for emergent or urgent surgery for any reason or any planned cardiac surgery within next 12 months
- Prior mitral valve leaflet surgery or any currently implanted prosthetic mitral valve, or any prior transcatheter mitral valve procedure
- Status 1 listing for heart transplant or prior orthotopic heart transplantation

Abbreviations: ACC/AHA, American College of Cardiology/American Heart Association; BNP, brain natriuretic peptide; CABG, coronary artery bypass grafting; CAD, coronary artery disease; COAPT, Cardiovascular Outcomes Assessment of the MitraClip Percutaneous Therapy for Heart Failure Patients with Functional Mitral Regurgitation; CRT, cardiac resynchronization therapy; CRT-D, cardiac resynchronization therapy with a device; HF, heart failure; MR, mitral regurgitation; NT-proBNP, N-terminal of the prohormone brain natriuretic peptide; NYHA, New York Heart Association; PCI, percutaneous coronary intervention; RV, right ventricular.

valve for FMR as an isolated operation has had mixed results at best. Current guidelines recommend operative intervention for FMR only with other cardiac operations, such as when other valve surgery or coronary bypass graft surgery is planned. What is needed to clarify the role of MitraClip for FMR? In the absence of randomized trials comparing surgery with past medical therapy, a randomized comparison of MitraClip with best medical therapy will be the only way to settle any questions regarding the role of MitraClip for FMR.

The Cardiovascular Outcomes Assessment of the MitraClip Percutaneous Therapy for Heart Failure Patients with Functional Mitral Regurgitation (COAPT) trial has been designed to address this question (Box 1). The COAPT trial is the first prospective, randomized, parallel-controlled clinical evaluation of the MitraClip device for the treatment of clinically significant FMR in patients who are not appropriate candidates for mitral valve surgery. The multicenter study will examine the safety and efficacy of the MitraClip device used in addition to standard care for MR and heart failure (device group) compared with treatment with standard care alone (control group). The trial will enroll 430 patients at up to 75 US sites. The long-term outcomes in FMR have historically not been studied with best medical therapy. The therapy for secondary MR is effectively heart failure therapy. Recently, an emphasis on guideline-directed medical therapy has led to a renewed interest in the use of medical therapy for FMR, and guideline-directed medical therapy will be the control arm for COAPT. Screening for the trial includes optimization of guideline-recommended medical therapy and an evaluation for CRT when appropriate. Only after patients are stable on guideline-directed medical therapy can they be randomized for the trial. The primary endpoint for efficacy is recurrent heart failure hospitalizations, and for safety a composite of single leaflet device attachment, device embolization, endocarditis requiring surgery, echocardiography core laboratory confirmed mitral stenosis requiring surgery, and any device-related complications requiring nonelective cardiovascular surgery at 12 months. Secondary endpoints for efficacy include MR severity at 12 month, changes in the 6-minute walk test, quality of life, LV end-diastolic volumes, and NYHA functional class I/II at 12 months. Secondary safety measures include the composite of all-cause death, stroke, myocardial infarction, or nonelective cardiovascular surgery for device related

complications at 30 days after the procedure in the MitraClip group.

Although the aggregate of nonrandomized global experience with MitraClip in FMR has been consistent in showing clear improvements in symptoms and favorable LV remodeling uncertainty remains regarding how MitraClip therapy will compare to best medical therapy. Thus, the COAPT trial will define the use of MitraClip in the foreseeable future.

REFERENCES

1. Nishimura RA, Otto CM, Bonow RO, et al. 2014 AHA/ACC guideline for the management of patients with valvular heart disease: a report of the American College of Cardiology/American Heart Association Task Force on Practice Guidelines. J Am Coll Cardiol 2014;63:e57–185.

2. Dayan V, Soca G, Cura L, et al. Similar survival after mitral valve replacement or repair for ischemic mitral regurgitation: a meta-analysis. Ann Thorac Surg 2014;97(3):758–65.

3. Feldman T, Young A. Percutaneous approaches to valve repair for mitral regurgitation. J Am Coll Cardiol 2014;63:2057–68.

4. St. Goar F. Development of percutaneous edge-to-edge repair: the MitraClip story. Chapter 6. In: Feldman T, St. Goar F, editors. Percutaneous mitral leaflet repair. London: Informa; 2012. p. 31–5.

5. Alfieri O, Maisano F, De Bonis M, et al. The double-orifice technique in mitral valve repair: a simple solution for complex problems. J Thorac Cardiovasc Surg 2001;122:674–81.

6. Feldman T, Foster E, Glower D, et al, For the EVEREST II Investigators. percutaneous repair or surgery for mitral regurgitation. N Engl J Med 2011;364: 1395–406.

7. Whitlow P, Feldman T, Pedersen W, et al, The EVEREST II High Risk Study. acute and 12 month results with catheter based mitral valve leaflet repair. J Am Coll Cardiol 2012;59:130–9.

8. Glower D, Kar S, Lim DS, et al. Percutaneous MitraClip device therapy for mitral regurgitation in 351 patients - high risk subset of the EVEREST II study. J Am Coll Cardiol 2014;64:172–81.

9. Philip F, Athappan G, Tuzcu EM, et al. MitraClip for severe symptomatic mitral regurgitation in patients at high surgical risk: a comprehensive systematic review. Catheter Cardiovasc Interv 2014; 84(4):581–90.

10. Schillinger W, Hünlich M, Baldus S, et al. Acute outcomes after MitraClip therapy in highly aged patients: results from the German TRAnscatheter Mitral valve Interventions (TRAMI) Registry. EuroIntervention 2013;9(1):84–90.

11. Franzen O, Baldus S, Rudolph V, et al. Acute outcomes of MitraClip therapy for mitral regurgitation in high-surgical-risk patients: emphasis on adverse valve morphology and severe left ventricular dysfunction. Eur Heart J 2010;31(11):1373–81.

12. Auricchio A, Schillinger W, Meyer S, et al, PERMIT-CARE Investigators. Correction of mitral regurgitation in nonresponders to cardiac resynchronization therapy by MitraClip improves symptoms and promotes reverse remodeling. J Am Coll Cardiol 2011;58(21):2183–9.

13. Seifert M, Schau T, Schoepp M, et al. MitraClip in CRT non-responders with severe mitral regurgitation. Int J Cardiol 2014;177(1):79–85.

14. Orban M, Braun D, Orban M, et al. Long-term outcome of patients with severe biventricular heart failure and severe mitral regurgitation after percutaneous edge-to-edge mitral valve repair. J Interv Cardiol 2015;28(2):164–71.

15. Attizzani GF, Ohno Y, Capodanno D, et al. Extended use of percutaneous edge-to-edge mitral valve repair beyond EVEREST (Endovascular Valve Edge-to-Edge Repair) criteria: 30-day and 12-month clinical and echocardiographic outcomes from the GRASP (Getting Reduction of Mitral Insufficiency by Percutaneous Clip Implantation) registry. JACC Cardiovasc Interv 2015;8(1 Pt A):74–82.

16. Feldman T, Salinger MH, Levisay JP, et al. MitraClip: path to approval and future directions: an overview of the key features, clinical use, and potential hurdles for this percutaneous mitral valve repair system. Cardiac Interventions Today 2014;1–4.

17. Lim DS, Reynolds MR, Feldman T, et al. Improved functional status and quality of life in prohibitive surgical risk patients with degenerative mitral regurgitation following transcatheter mitral valve repair with the MitraClip system. J Am Coll Cardiol 2014;64:182–92.

Coronary Sinus-Based Approach to Mitral Regurgitation

 CrossMark

Steven L. Goldberg, MD[a,b,*],
Christoph Hammerstingl, MD[c]

KEYWORDS

- Mitral regurgitation • Coronary sinus • Carillon device

KEY POINTS

- Use of the Carillon device in the coronary sinus has been shown to reduce functional mitral regurgitation, and improve symptoms in patients with congestive heart failure.
- The Carillon device has been associated with a low rate of major adverse events.
- A double blind randomized trial is currently ongoing comparing the Carillon device against optimal medical therapy.

The venous drainage of the heart empties into the great cardiac vein, which becomes the coronary sinus midway between the vein's origin at the anterior interventricular vein and the coronary sinus ostium where it drains into the right atrium. Frequently there is a venous valve at this midportion, the valve of Vieussens, which demarcates the differentiation where the great cardiac vein becomes the coronary sinus. This venous structure lies about 1 cm above the posterior mitral annulus on the left atrial size and passes parallel to the annulus, extending from approximately commissure to commissure. Secondary or functional mitral regurgitation (FMR) occurs when the mitral leaflets are effectively normal; however, cardiomyopathy-induced annular dilation and/or tethering of the mitral valve affects its competence. The relationship between the great cardiac vein and coronary sinus (henceforth referred to as the coronary sinus) has been used to place devices capable of providing a cinching force on the posterior annulus of the mitral annulus. Theoretically, this force on the mitral annulus may be helpful in reducing secondary mitral regurgitation by reducing annular size.

Based on echo studies, FMR affects 45% to 100% (average 60%) of patients with congestive heart failure, with 24% to 58% (average 40%) having more than mild FMR.[1–7] This suggests that the prevalence of FMR is vast, affecting several-fold more individuals than aortic stenosis. It is, therefore, the most common dysfunctional valvular heart disease, even though the intrinsic components of the valve structure itself are normal. The presence of FMR is clinically important because patients with congestive heart failure who have FMR have a variety of worse clinical outcomes and associated high-risk features. Compared with patients without FMR, patients with FMR have a higher risk of mortality,[1–4,7] poorer exercise performance[3,8] and functional class,[1–4] a higher prevalence of tricuspid regurgitation,[1,4] worsened hemodynamic parameters,[3] and larger left atrial and ventricular chamber sizes.[6,8] These parameters

---

Disclosures: S.L. Goldberg receives consultancy payments and stock options from Cardiac Dimensions, Inc. C. Hammerstingl receives payments for consultancy work from Cardiac Dimensions, Inc.
[a] Rocky Mountain Heart & Lung, Kalispell Regional Medical Center, 350 Heritage Way, Suite 2100, Kalispell, MT 59901, USA; [b] Cardiac Dimensions, Inc, 5540 Lake Washington Boulevard NE, Kirkland, WA 98033, USA; [c] Heart Center University of Bonn, Sigmund Freud Strasse 25, Bonn 53125, Germany
* Corresponding author. Rocky Mountain Heart & Lung, Kalispell Regional Medical Center, 350 Heritage Way, Suite 2100, Kalispell, MT 59901.
E-mail address: stevgold99@gmail.com

are all associated with worse clinical outcomes.[9] Therefore, there has been interest in finding techniques capable of modifying the distortion, dilation, and/or tethering of the mitral annulus as a means to reduce the mitral valve dysfunction and associated clinical impact of that dysfunction. Surgical annular reduction has been used but its value has not been confirmed. It is currently a 2b American College of Cardiology/American Heart Association (AHA/ACC) recommendation for patients not otherwise undergoing cardiac surgery and 2a for patients referred for other cardiac surgery.[10,11] MitraClip (Abbott Laboratories, Abbott Park, Illinois) is widely used to treat FMR in certain countries. Randomized trials evaluating the effectiveness of this therapy to treat FMR are ongoing in the United States and elsewhere.[12]

The cinching force, potentially applicable to the posterior annulus of the mitral valve by a device inside the coronary sinus, has been considered as a possible avenue to reduce mitral annular dimensions and, potentially, the severity of FMR and the associated clinical impact. Several devices have been proposed and tested inside the coronary sinus with the intention of cinching the mitral valve, although only one is currently being implanted in humans. Cerclage has been tested in animals. It consists of a wire inside the coronary sinus, encircles the mitral annulus, and then exits into the right atrium or right ventricle. Because the circumflex coronary artery typically courses in the left atrial atrioventricular groove, as well as in the coronary sinus, a proprietary device to create a bridge over the coronary artery has been developed that prevents coronary artery compression from the constricting force of the wire inside the coronary sinus.[13] This therapy has not yet been attempted in humans.

Several other devices have had evaluation in humans. The Ample PS3 system, now called the ARTO System (MVRx, Belmont, California), consists of an anchor placed in the coronary sinus, which is connected to an interatrial septal occluder by means of a connecting bridge, which can be tensioned, reducing the anterior-posterior mitral annular diameter.[14] Phase I clinical trials with the ARTO System are ongoing. The MONARC (Edwards LifeSciences, Irvine, California) device, no longer in active investigation, consisted of 2 self-expanding stents with a connecting segment. The distal stent was placed in the anterior-interventricular vein and the proximal one in the coronary sinus ostium. The connecting segment had self-absorbing spacers, which allowed a slowly developing

shortening of this segment, applying a gradual cinching of the system. This gradual shortening was intended to minimize the impact of the cinching force on the circumflex coronary artery; however, rare late circumflex coronary artery compression and resultant myocardial infarctions were seen.[15] Of note, the distal stent was placed in the anterior interventricular vein, which provided strong anchoring characteristics but likely led to greater force applied to circumflex coronary arteries than a device completely in the great cardiac vein. A small, unpublished, safety and efficacy study was completed that suggested that the proof of concept of a coronary sinus approach was supported, with a reported reduction of mitral regurgitation.[15] The Viacor (Viacor, Inc. Wilmington, MA) device consisted of a catheter delivered inside the coronary sinus, into which 1 to 3 stiffening bars could be delivered to provide a compression force on the posterior annulus. This device was evaluated in an unpublished safety and efficacy study, wherein reportedly a reduction in mitral regurgitation was seen with this device.[16,17] However, rare extrusions of the catheter from the coronary sinus were also observed, leading to clinically meaningful perforations, and subsequent studies were discontinued.[18] In addition, this device was associated with coronary artery compression, exacerbated by the placement of the distal aspect of the device in the anterior interventricular vein, rather than the great cardiac vein. However, the removability of the stiffening rods allowed for successful removal of the tension and return of normal coronary artery flow,[19] a characteristic shared by the Carillon device.

The Carillon Mitral Contour System (Cardiac Dimensions, Inc, Kirkland, WA) is a nitinol-based device with 2 self-expanding anchors. Coronary sinus access is obtained via a 9 French catheter in the right internal jugular vein. The distal anchor is delivered and locked into the distal great cardiac vein, just before the anterior interventricular vein. Manual tension is applied to the system and a proximal anchor is delivered and locked. Both anchors are sized based on quantitative measurements of venous dimensions. Until released, the device may be recaptured and removed. This may be done if there is external compression of the circumflex or distal branch of the right coronary artery, if there is insufficient reduction in mitral regurgitation, or if the device is not placed in its intended location. With access of the coronary sinus, the procedure is simple and quick, with the entire procedure taking less than 45 minutes (**Fig. 1**).

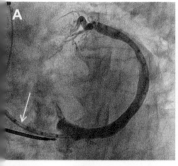
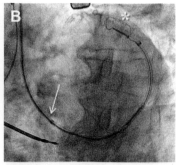
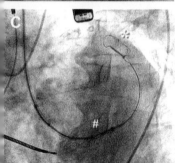
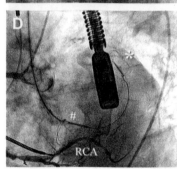

Fig. 1. Procedural steps of the device implantation. (*A*) Angiogram of the coronary sinus with the marker catheter in place (*arrow*). (*B*) Placement of the distal anchor (*asterisk*) via the device sheath (*arrow*). (*C*) Deployment of the proximal anchor (*hash*). (*D*) Final assessment of coronary flow under tension and foreshortening of the coronary sinus with both anchors in place (*asterisk, hash*). RCA, right coronary artery.

Three safety and efficacy studies were carried out in Europe: AMADEUS (CARILLON Mitral Annuloplasty Device European Union Study), TITAN, and TITAN II.[20,21] TITAN II is currently awaiting publication. The studies were similar in their entry requirements. All subjects had to have symptomatic congestive heart failure, New York Heart Association classification (NYHA) 2 to 4, 6 minute walk test (6 MWT) 150 to 450 m, 2+ or greater FMR, depressed left ventricular function (ejection fraction <40%), and dilated left ventricle (left ventricular end-diastolic diameter >55 mm). The studies differed in the use of minor device modifications between the studies. Specifically, a twist was added to the distal anchor in AMADEUS to address the tendency of the anchor to slip when tension was applied. A twist was added to the proximal anchor for the TITAN study for theoretic reasons (to minimize the possibility of proximal anchor slipping). In this study, several proximal anchors fractured, which were clinically silent with no complications or loss of efficacy. A stress analysis of the device (specifically the proximal anchor) revealed an area of high strain where the fractures occurred. This led to some minor modifications to reduce the strain and this modified device was used in TITAN II.

Each of the studies demonstrated a low incidence of major adverse events out to 30 days and no events were deemed to be device-related by independent safety and monitoring boards.

There was clinical benefit in each trial, with a consistent 1-grade improvement in NYHA class and approximately 100 m 6 MWT increase seen in all 3 trials. These benefits were seen immediately and demonstrated durability for 2 years (evaluated for 6 MWT) and 4 years (for NYHA class).

Echocardiographic improvements were also seen (**Fig. 2**). Significant reductions in quantitative parameters of mitral regurgitation were seen in subjects with implants compared with baseline in the TITAN study. Similar trends were seen in AMADEUS and TITAN II. Interestingly, in these studies, there was evidence of the mitral regurgitation (MR) improving with time, with less MR in subjects with implants at 12 months than at 1 or 6 months. In addition to improvements in MR, reductions in left ventricular dimensions were seen, most notably in TITAN, suggesting the improvement in MR led to favorable ventricular remodeling.

The TITAN trial had a pseudo-control group of subjects who had the device placed but then removed, either due to temporary coronary artery compression or inadequate reduction in acute myocardial infarction. These subjects did not show improvements in any of the clinical or echocardiographic parameters described previously.

Coronary artery compression limited permanent implantation of the Carillon device in 10% to 15% of subjects in these trials. In AMADEUS, there were 3 instances of cardiac enzyme

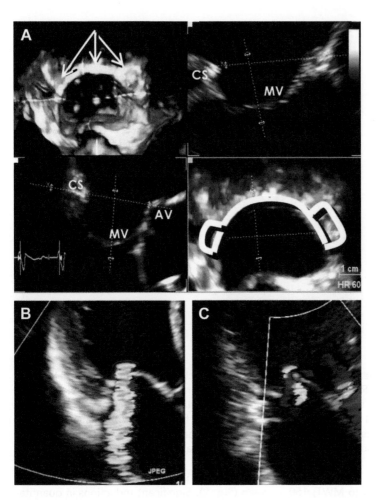

Fig. 2. Echocardiography after device placement. (A) Three-dimensional enface view of the mitral annulus demonstrating proper device placement (arrows) encircling most of the posterior part of the annulus. (B) MR before device implantation and (C) after 3 months of follow-up. AV, aortic valve; CS, coronary sinus; MV, mitral valve.

elevations postprocedure but no acute or long-term device-related myocardial infarctions were otherwise seen and no cases in either of the other 2 trials. This is in contrast to the previously mentioned MONARC coronary sinus-based device. Important differences between the MONARC and Carillon devices related to coronary artery compromise include the ability to recapture the Carillon device immediately if angiographic compression is visualized. Additionally, the placement of the Carillon distal anchor in the great cardiac vein, rather than the anterior interventricular vein, is important because an anchoring system in the anterior interventricular vein crosses more arteries and applies greater force to those arteries. Finally, the MONARC device developed its cinching force over time, potentially leading to progressive coronary artery compression.

As mentioned previously, several Carillon devices developed fractures at a specific location in the proximal anchor in the TITAN study. This

seemed to be adequately addressed with the modification used in the TITAN study. As mentioned, the fractures in TITAN did not cause complications or diminish the effectiveness of the device.

A mechanistic, double-blind randomized trial, REDUCE FMR, has been initiated in Europe and Australia. In this study, subjects will be randomized on the table to device (with continued optimal medical therapy) or to optimal medical therapy alone, and followed for 1 year looking for reduction in regurgitant volume. Secondary endpoints to be evaluated include impact on 6 MWT and NYHA class (more meaningful given the double-blind nature of the study), as well as heart failure hospitalizations.

Another small, investigator-driven pilot study, CLINCH (Clip versus Cinch), is being done in Germany comparing Carillon to MitraClip, with a built-in crossover arm.

Finally, the Carillon device has received a conformité européene (CE) mark approval for sale in

Europe and is being commercially implemented in certain countries.

Procedural Steps

- The procedure can be done with transthoracic or transesophageal echo monitoring, using conscious sedation or general anesthesia.
- Arterial access is obtained for coronary artery imaging.
- Venous access in the right internal jugular vein is obtained, with placement of a 9 French sheath.
- Right and left coronary artery angiography is performed. During left coronary artery angiography, prolonged imaging for the venous phase is performed to visualize the coronary sinus and great cardiac vein. This allows for a rough assessment of suitability of the vein and provides a roadmap for access. Left anterior oblique caudal or cranial is most useful.
- Coronary sinus access is obtained with the 9 French delivery catheter.
- A marker catheter, which has radiopaque markers at each centimeter, is inserted into the delivery catheter.
- Left coronary artery angiography is performed in the right and left anterior oblique with caudal angulation views to assess the relationship between the circumflex coronary artery and the coronary vein.
- Venography is performed in the same views (**Fig. 3**).
- Using the marker catheter as a scaling device, measurements are made of the vein at the anticipated site of the distal and proximal anchors. An assessment of the usable vein length is also made (**Fig. 4**).
- With the imaging system in the same left anterior oblique with caudal angulation, the active fluoroscopy screen is marked with an erasable marker at the intended location of the distal anchor. Another mark is made at the intended location of the proximal anchor, after the desired tension is applied (**Fig. 5**).
- The marker catheter is removed. Each Carillon device (**Fig. 6**) is prepackaged in a cartridge connected to a cable, which is, in turn, connected to a delivery handle with 3 rotating knobs (**Fig. 7**). The cartridge is attached to the delivery catheter and the cable is advanced until

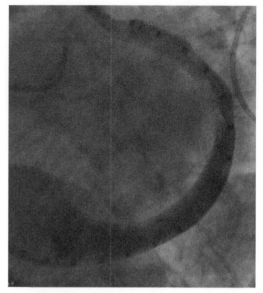

Fig. 3. Preprocedural venogram of the great cardiac vein and coronary sinus.

the cartridge can be attached to the delivery handle.

- The first knob is then rotated in the direction of the dark arrow. Under fluoroscopy, this causes the distal anchor to be extruded out of the delivery catheter (**Fig. 8**). To compensate for this forward motion, the operator gently pulls back on the delivery catheter to have the distal aspect of the distal anchor land at the level of the mark on the screen.
- After the distal anchor is seen to open, as it is unsheathed, the control knob is rotated in the opposite direction. This allows for locking of the device, by pushing the delivery catheter against an eyelet, which can be advanced over a lock bump.

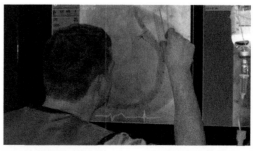

Fig. 4. Planning the location of the distal and proximal anchors of the device.

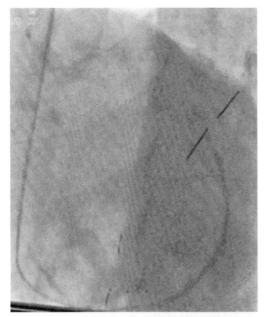

Fig. 5. The distal (top of screen) and proximal (bottom of screen) anchor locations have been marked using an erasable marker on the fluoroscopy screen.

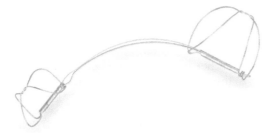

Fig. 6. The Carillon device.

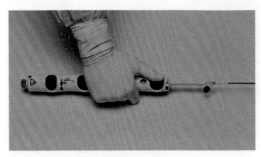

Fig. 7. The Carillon delivery system.

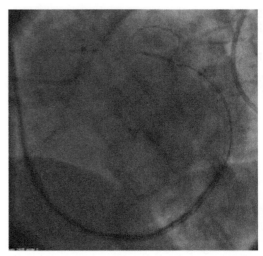

Fig. 8. The distal anchor (top of screen) being extruded from the delivery catheter.

- Tension is then applied to the delivery catheter until the proximal aspect of the proximal anchor crimp tube is seen to align with the mark on the fluoroscopy screen as the preferred location of the proximal anchor, typically near the ostium of the coronary sinus.
- Left coronary angiography is then performed. If there is no compromise of the coronary artery, the proximal anchor may then be placed (Fig. 9).

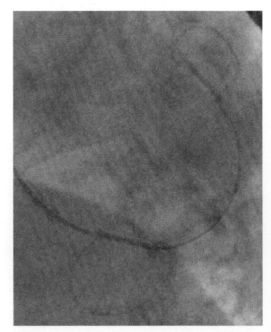

Fig. 9. The proximal anchor (bottom of screen) after delivery.

- To place the proximal anchor, the first control knob is again rotated in the direction of the dark arrow, which causes continued unsheathing of the device.
- After the first control knob rotation comes to a stop, the operator switches to the second control knob, which again is rotated in the direction of the dark arrow. This causes a pusher inside the delivery system to push the proximal anchor out and to induce locking of the anchor, again with a loop advancing over a lock bump.
- Echocardiographic assessment may be done at this point to look for the impact on mitral regurgitation.
- Right coronary angiography is done because, rarely, the proximal anchor can impinge on a long branch of the posterolateral marginal branch.
- If there is reason to recapture the device, it can be done at any point until the device is released. Possible reasons for recapture include coronary artery compression, insufficient reduction in mitral regurgitation, slipping of the distal anchor during tensioning, improper placement of the device, or distorted appearance of the anchors.
- The proximal anchor is recaptured by turning the first knob away from the dark arrow, while gently compressing the delivery catheter with the left hand, maintaining appropriate tension. After the proximal anchor is recaptured, gentle compression is applied to the delivery catheter to approximate the curvature of the vein in its resting state.
- Recapture, or resheathing, of the distal anchor is then performed by rotating the first knob away from the dark arrow and gently advancing the delivery catheter with the left hand.
- A new device may be attempted if deemed appropriate.
- If recapturing of the device is not necessary and the delivered device is deemed acceptable, release of the device is then performed. The red safety cap on the back of the delivery handle is removed and the third knob is rotated in the direction of the dark arrow until the device is released. The procedure is then complete.

SUMMARY

Although several devices use the close relationship of the coronary sinus and posterior annulus of the mitral valve to provide a cinching force on the mitral valve, only the Carillon device is implanted in patients. The initial studies evaluating this device have been favorable and an ongoing randomized trial is being done to confirm those favorable findings.

REFERENCES

1. Blondheim DS, Jacobs LE, Kotler MN, et al. Dilated cardiomyopathy with mitral regurgitation: decreased survival despite a low frequency of left ventricular thrombus. Am Heart J 1991;122:763–71.
2. Cioffi G, Tarantini L, De Feo S, et al. Functional mitral regurgitation predicts 1-year mortality in elderly patients with systolic chronic heart failure. Eur J Heart Fail 2005;7:1112–7.
3. Junker A, Thayssen P, Nielsen B, et al. The hemodynamic and prognostic significance of echo-Doppler-proven mitral regurgitation in patients with dilated cardiomyopathy. Cardiology 1993;83: 14–20.
4. Koelling TM, Aaronson KD, Cody RJ, et al. Prognostic significance of mitral regurgitation and tricuspid regurgitation in patients with left ventricular systolic dysfunction. Am Heart J 2002;144:524–9.
5. Patel AR, Mochizuki Y, Yao J, et al. Mitral regurgitation: comprehensive assessment by echocardiography. Echocardiography 2000;17:275–83.
6. Strauss RH, Stevenson LW, Dadourian BA, et al. Predictability of mitral regurgitation detected by Doppler echocardiography in patients referred for cardiac transplantation. Am J Cardiol 1987;59: 892–4.
7. Trichon BH, Felker GM, Shaw LK, et al. Relation of frequency and severity of mitral regurgitation to survival among patients with left ventricular systolic dysfunction and heart failure. Am J Cardiol 2003;91: 538–43.
8. Tada H, Tamai J, Takaki H, et al. Mild mitral regurgitation reduces exercise capacity in patients with idiopathic dilated cardiomyopathy. Int J Cardiol 1997;58:41–5.
9. Lancellotti P, Gérard PL, Piérard LA. Long-term outcome of patients with heart failure and dynamic functional mitral regurgitation. Eur Heart J 2005;26: 1528–32.
10. Nishimura RA, Otto CM, Bonow RO, et al, American College of Cardiology/American Heart Association Task Force on Practice Guidelines. 2014 AHA/ACC guideline for the management of patients with valvular heart disease: a report of the American College of Cardiology/American Heart Association Task Force on Practice Guidelines. J Am Coll Cardiol 2014;63:e57–185.
11. Wu AH, Aaronson KD, Bolling SF, et al. Impact of mitral valve annuloplasty on mortality risk in

patients with mitral regurgitation and left ventricular systolic dysfunction. J Am Coll Cardiol 2005;45: 381–7.

12. Asgar AW, Mack MJ, Stone GW. Secondary mitral regurgitation in heart failure: pathophysiology, prognosis, and therapeutic considerations. J Am Coll Cardiol 2015;65:1231–48.

13. Kim JH, Kocaturk O, Ozturk C, et al. Mitral cerclage annuloplasty, a novel transcatheter treatment for secondary mitral valve regurgitation: initial results in swine. J Am Coll Cardiol 2009;54:638–51.

14. Rogers JH, Macoviak JA, Rahdert DA, et al. Percutaneous septal sinus shortening: a novel procedure for the treatment of functional mitral regurgitation. Circulation 2006;113:2329–34.

15. Harnek J, Webb JG, Kuck KH, et al. Transcatheter implantation of the MONARC coronary sinus device for mitral regurgitation: 1-year results from the EVOLUTION phase I study (Clinical Evaluation of the Edwards Lifesciences Percutaneous Mitral Annuloplasty System for the Treatment of Mitral Regurgitation). JACC Cardiovasc Interv 2011;4: 115–22.

16. Bertrand OF, Philippon F, St Pierre A, et al. Percutaneous mitral valve annuloplasty for functional mitral regurgitation: acute results of the first patient treated with the Viacor permanent device and future perspectives. Cardiovasc Revasc Med 2010; 11:265.e1–8.

17. Sack S, Kahlert P, Bilodeau L, et al. Percutaneous transvenous mitral annuloplasty: initial human experience with a novel coronary sinus implant device. Circ Cardiovasc Interv 2009;2:277–84.

18. Machaalany J, St-Pierre A, Senechal M, et al. Fatal late migration of viacor percutaneous transvenous mitral annuloplasty device resulting in distal coronary venous perforation. Can J Cardiol 2013;29: 130.e1–4.

19. Sponga S, Bertrand OF, Philippon F, et al. Reversible circumflex coronary artery occlusion during percutaneous transvenous mitral annuloplasty with the Viacor system. J Am Coll Cardiol 2012; 59:288.

20. Schofer J, Siminiak T, Haude M, et al. Percutaneous mitral annuloplasty for functional mitral regurgitation: results of the CARILLON Mitral Annuloplasty Device European Union Study. Circulation 2009; 120:326–33.

21. Siminiak T, Wu JC, Haude M, et al. Treatment of functional mitral regurgitation by percutaneous annuloplasty: results of the TITAN Trial. Eur J Heart Fail 2012;14:931–8.

Percutaneous Mitral Annuloplasty

Maurizio Taramasso, MD[a], Azeem Latib, MD[b],*

KEYWORDS

- Mitral valve • Functional mitral regurgitation • Percutaneous annuloplasty • Direct annuloplasty
- Transcatheter mitral valve intervention

KEY POINTS

- Transcatheter annuloplasty has the potential to improve outcomes and to increase therapeutic options for patients with mitral regurgitation (MR) who are at high-risk for surgical repair.
- Different catheter-based devices have made use of the coronary sinus (CS) to achieve indirect annuloplasty, whereas other devices achieve direct annuloplasty or ventriculoplasty.
- Transcatheter mitral annuloplasty preserves the native valve anatomy, thus keeping the option for future valve treatment open.
- In patients who have degenerative MR, transcatheter annuloplasty may represent an adjunct therapy, in combination with leaflet repair, to achieve better acute results and improve repair durability.
- In patients who have functional MR and favorable anatomy, annuloplasty might represent a stand-alone procedure.

INTRODUCTION

Percutaneous mitral valve therapies are emerging as an alternative option for high-risk patients who are not good candidates for conventional open-heart surgery. In recent years, multiple technologies and diversified approaches have been developed and are currently under clinical study or in preclinical development.[1]

Conventionally, these devices are classified according to the anatomic and pathophysiological addressed target: indirect and direct annuloplasty, leaflet and chordal repair procedures, or left ventricular (LV) remodeling devices. This article focuses on transcatheter mitral annuloplasty devices, describes the different technologies, and reports on the initial clinical and preclinical experiences.

THE BACKGROUND: SURGICAL ANNULOPLASTY

Mitral annuloplasty is mostly performed during conventional mitral surgery to restore the normal ratio between the leaflet surface area and the annular area and to improve leaflet coaptation. Moreover, it has been shown that mitral annuloplasty prevents progressive annular dilatation and consequent recurrent mitral regurgitation (MR) after surgery[2–4] and reduces stress forces acting on the valve leaflet,[5,6] which may prevent suture dehiscence.

Although suture annuloplasty is rarely performed nowadays, implantation of a prosthetic mitral ring is currently the gold standard surgical technique for mitral annuloplasty.[7–10] Different shaped mitral rings have been developed for different types of MR,[11,12] and the choice of

---

[a] Department of Cardiac Surgery, Herz-Gefäss Chirurgie, UniversitätsSpital Zürich, Rämistrasse 100, 8091, Zürich, Switzerland; [b] Interventional Cardiology Unit, EMO-GVM Centro Cuore Columbus, San Raffaele Scientific Institute, Via Buonarroti 48, Milan 20145, Italy
* Corresponding author.
E-mail address: info@emocolumbus.it

Intervent Cardiol Clin 5 (2016) 101–107
http://dx.doi.org/10.1016/j.iccl.2015.08.009
2211-7458/16/$ – see front matter © 2016 Elsevier Inc. All rights reserved.

the device usually depends on the preference and experience of the surgeon and on the MR type (complete or incomplete; rigid, semi-rigid or flexible).

In the context of degenerative MR (DMR), in which the mitral leaflets are intrinsically diseased, annuloplasty is usually performed in association with leaflet repair techniques to reduce MR recurrence due to further annular dilatation.[4] In functional MR (FMR), undersized annuloplasty is effectively performed as a stand-alone procedure and it is associated with satisfactory results when proper patient selection is carried out.[13–18] Undersized annuloplasty is able to reduce the septolateral diameter of the mitral annulus, therefore forcing leaflet coaptation, balancing the coaptation defect due to leaflet tethering.[19]

Long-term durability is a major concern of undersized annuloplasty in FMR, with an overall recurrence of significant MR ranging from 10% to 30% at 1 year. Proper patient selection based on preoperative echocardiography is the major determinant of long-term outcomes.[13,14,20–24] The main determinants of failure after undersized annuloplasty in FMR are the following[25]:

- Mild annular dilatation
- Complex multiple regurgitant jets
- Advanced LV remodeling
- Excessive tethering (coaptation depth >1.5 cm)
- Posterior mitral leaflet angle greater than 45°
- Distal anterior mitral leaflet angle greater than 25°
- Systolic tenting area greater than 2.5 cm^2
- End-systolic interpapillary muscle distance greater than 20 mm
- Systolic specificity index greater than 0.7.

THE CLINICAL NEED FOR TRANSCATHETER MITRAL ANNULOPLASTY

The unavailability of a reliable annuloplasty device has reduced the overall clinical applicability for transcatheter mitral interventions. Transcatheter annuloplasty has the potential to improve outcomes and to increase therapeutic options. As soon as annuloplasty devices become clinically available, percutaneous techniques may become a true alternative to surgery in selected patients.

Transcatheter edge-to-edge repair with the MitraClip system (Abbott Vascular Inc, Menlo, CA, USA) is currently the most advanced technology available for clinical use, with a proven safety and efficacy profile in selected patients with either FMR or DMR.[26–28] Improvements of symptoms, quality of life, and MR reduction have been observed in most cases. However, about 20% of patients do not respond as expected to MitraClip therapy. Residual MR after the procedure is often due to the concomitant annular dilatation, which is not addressed by the MitraClip.[26,29]

Surgical experience has shown that long-term results of surgical edge-to-edge in the absence of annuloplasty are suboptimal.[30] Therefore, the absence of mitral annuloplasty is a major concern regarding the long-term durability of MitraClip therapy. The combination of transcatheter annuloplasty and MitraClip has the potential to improve durability and, therefore, expand the indication toward a lower risk population.

The absence of transcatheter annuloplasty devices is also limiting the global number of patients who could benefit from a less invasive transcatheter treatment. Up to 30% of patients screened for MitraClip are refused due to anatomic ineligibility, including annular dilatation,[31] suggesting that there is a clinical need for a different transcatheter mitral repair approach to address annular dilatation. Another important limitation of MitraClip is that it removes future therapeutic options for transcatheter mitral valve replacement. One of the most appealing features of transcatheter mitral annuloplasty is that this approach preserves the native valve anatomy, thus keeping the option for future valve treatment open. In fact, some of the annuloplasty devices may actually serve as a dock or anchoring zone for the implantation of commercially available transcatheter aortic valves.

DESCRIPTION OF ANNULOPLASTY DEVICES AND PRELIMINARY RESULTS

Different catheter-based devices have made use of the CS to achieve indirect annuloplasty, whereas other devices achieve direct annuloplasty or ventriculoplasty.

Indirect Annuloplasty
The indirect annuloplasty approach is based on the anatomic proximity of the CS to the posterior mitral annulus. The CS encircles about two-thirds of the mitral annulus and can be used as a route to push the posterior annulus toward the anterior, reducing the septolateral diameter and forcing leaflet coaptation. The cannulation of the CS is easy, reproducible,

and not technically demanding; therefore this approach is particularly appealing.

Early attempts to remodel the mitral annulus have been based on CS annuloplasty[32–34] but initial results have been mixed, mainly due to suboptimal efficacy and the risk of delayed complications, including coronary occlusion.[32,35,36]

The Carillon Mitral Contour System (Cardiac Dimension, Inc, Kirkland, WA, USA) is the only technology still using this approach. It obtained Conformité Européenne (CE) mark in 2011 and, therefore, is commercially available in Europe. The Transcatheter Implantation of Carillon Mitral Annuloplasty Device (TITAN) trial, which evaluated the clinical impact of the Carillon in heart failure subjects with significant FMR, showed a significant reduction in FMR grade with a reduction in LV diastolic and systolic volumes. Treated subjects were compared with a pseudo-control group consisting of subjects without implants. Functional and performance status significantly improved in the treated subjects. Late results showed that CS annuloplasty was associated with delayed reverse LV remodeling and clinical improvements up to 24 months even in subjects in whom an acute response was not observed.[37] The upcoming REDUCE (Safety and Efficacy of the CARILLON Mitral Contour System in Reducing Functional Mitral Regurgitation Associated eith Heart Failure) randomized trial will compare the Carillon device to optimal medical therapy in 120 heart failure subjects with FMR. The first subject was enrolled in June 2015.

Although clinical benefits have been observed, this approach may not be applicable or effective in all patients with FMR because the CS and mitral annulus are not coplanar and because of the risk of coronary artery compression. However, the procedure is easy to perform, can be done under local anesthesia in centers without on-site cardiac surgery, and is very safe. The absence of a surgical basis for the CS approach may be a concern as regards the long-term outcomes of this procedure.

Direct Annuloplasty

Direct mitral valve annuloplasty is thus far the most promising approach for transcatheter mitral valve annuloplasty because it closely reproduces the conventional surgical approach. Various technologies are under clinical and preclinical investigation.

The Valtech Cardioband

The Valtech Cardioband (ValtechCardio, Inc, Or Yehuda, Israel) is the closest transcatheter device to a surgical ring[38] (**Fig. 1**). It is delivered from a transseptal approach and the implant is performed on the atrial side of the mitral annulus. An incomplete adjustable surgical-like Dacron band is implanted from commissure to commissure, under live echo and fluoroscopic guidance, using multiple anchor elements. The interaction with cardiac function and the hemodynamic impact are minimal. After implantation, the Cardioband length may be shortened on the beating heart under live echo guidance to improve leaflet coaptation and reduce MR. The CE Mark Trial is currently enrolling high-risk subjects with FMR. Initial clinical experiences are promising, confirming the feasibility and safety of the Cardioband implantation. Preliminary data achieved in 40 symptomatic subjects with FMR from the CE Mark Trial have been recently reported (Vahanian A. *Cardioband: procedure; insights from CT planning, and CE Mark Trial results*. Presented at the TVT Conference. Chicago, June 4, 2015) showing that Cardioband

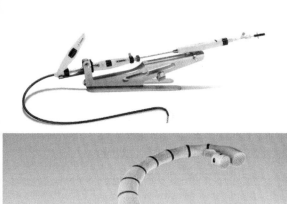

Fig. 1. The Valtech transseptal delivery system (*upper panel*) and adjustable Dacron band (*lower panel*). (*Courtesy of* Valtech Cardio, Or Yehuda, Israel; with permission.)

implant is associated with significant septolateral annular dimension reduction (20% on average) and increased leaflet coaptation surface. Acute significant MR reduction was achieved in more than 95% of the subjects and 85% of the subjects had MR greater than or equal to 2+ at 6 months. Thirty-day mortality was 5% (2 out of 40 subjects), with a very low incidence of major events, suggesting the procedure is safe even in high-risk patients. The main concern regarding this procedure will be the clinical applicability in unselected FMR patients when the device is commercialized and the relatively steep learning curve.

The Mitralign System

The Mitralign system (Mitralign, Inc, Tewksbury, MA, USA) is designed to perform selective plication of the mitral annulus (in the P1 and P3 annular segments) by deploying pairs of transannular pledgets that are delivered by a transfemoral retrograde approach through the mitral annulus[39] (Fig. 2). The procedure is performed under live echo and fluoroscopic guidance. The results of the CE Mark Trial have been recently reported in 51 high-risk subjects with FMR. Thirty-day mortality was 7.8%; survival at 6 months was 88% with an 80% of freedom from valve intervention. Significant improvements in MR severity, reduction in annular dimensions, and significant LV remodeling were demonstrated at 6 months (Schofer J. *Mitralign procedure and results of the CE Mark Trial.* Presented at the TVT Conference. Chicago, June 4, 2015). Results from the study also confirmed that 2 pairs of pledgets

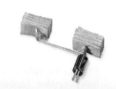
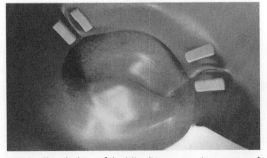

Fig. 2. The pledget of the Mitralign system (*upper panel*) and image showing 2 pairs of pledgets implanted in the mitral annulus (*lower panel*). (*Courtesy of* Mitralign Inc, Tewksbury, MA; with permission.)

were more effective in reducing MR than a single pair of pledgets. The procedure was also safe with no procedure-related events.

The Accucinch System

The Accucinch system (Guided Delivery Systems, Inc, Santa Clara, CA, USA) is another direct annuloplasty device using the retrograde transventricular approach. A series of anchors are implanted in the subannular space beneath the MV in the base of the LV (Fig. 3) and, because anchors are not directly placed in the annulus, this procedure may best be described as ventriculoplasty rather than annuloplasty. The anchors are connected by a nitinol wire in which tethering the cord under echo guidance cinches the basal LV and mitral annulus. A peculiar aspect of the Accucinch System is that it also causes remodeling of the basal portion of the LV, promoting papillary muscle approximation. The feasibility and the safety of the device has been shown in 18 subjects; 5 were converted to surgery and no 30- day deaths occurred. In the cases of the 4 most recent subjects of this small series, about 40% of reduction of MR (quantified as regurgitant volume and effective regurgitant area) and a clinical improvement were observed (Kleber F. *Basal ventriculoplasty: guided delivery systems: Accucinch design iterations and clinical results.* Presented at the TCT Conference. San Francisco, October 28, 2013). After these promising initial clinical data, no further updates have been provided to date.

Cardiac Implants Mitral Restriction Ring

Cardiac Implants Mitral Restriction Ring (Cardiac Implant Solutions LLC, Jacksonville, FL, USA) is another direct annuloplasty device delivered via the transseptal route (similarly to the Cardioband), which is currently under preclinical investigation (35 acute and chronic animal implants reported so far). It allows the implantation of a complete adjustable mitral ring with an internal cinching wire on the atrial annular side by means of multiple anchor elements. The implantable actuator is designed to enable noninvasive chronic progressive cinching also at follow-up, following the completion of tissue healing. In case of MR recurrence, the complete mitral ring may serve as support for a transcatheter valve-in-ring implantation. Feasibility has been reported in animal models (Kuck KH. *Progressive mitral ring annuloplasty and mitral valve replacement. Based on single shot percutaneous implantation of complete circumferential ring.*

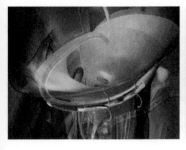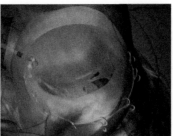

Fig. 3. The Accucinch anchor delivery catheter (*left panel*) and image showing the fully implanted device before cinching (*right panel*). (*Courtesy of* Guided Delivery Systems, Santa Clara, CA; with permission.)

Presented at the TCT Conference. San Francisco, September 14, 2014).

The Valcare Medical AMEND

The Valcare Medical AMEND (Valcare Medical, Herzlyia Pituach, Israel) is a complete, semirigid, D-shaped mitral ring, which is implanted on the atrial side of the mitral annulus by means of 12 anchors, through transapical access. An acute animal study on 40 adult pigs showed feasibility of the procedure, with a 20% to 25% reduction of the septolateral annular dimension after the implantation. Also, this device can potentially serve as a platform for future valve in ring implantation in case of MR recurrence (Meerkin D. *AMEND. The mitral solution from Valcare.* Presented at the EuroPCR Conference. Paris, May 18, 2015).

Other Annular Repair Techniques

Beyond indirect CS annuloplasty and direct annuloplasty, other methods have been attempted to remodel the mitral annulus, including external compression of atrioventricular groove,[40] implantation of cinching devices,[41] and application of RF or US energy sources to shrink the annular collagen.[42,43] Reproducibility, efficacy and safety of these appealing technologies needs to be still proved because they are based on completely novel concepts, without a validated and reproducible surgical or preclinical background.

SUMMARY

The precise clinical role of transcatheter mitral annuloplasty is still not yet well established because it is a new therapeutic approach and clinical results are still limited. However, based on the preliminary results of the different technologies and on the lessons learned from surgery, it is possible to try to define what the clinical role of this therapy will be:

- In DMR patients, annuloplasty may represent an adjunctive therapy in combination with leaflet repair, to achieve better acute results and improve repair durability.
- In FMR patients, annuloplasty might represent a stand-alone procedure in patients with favorable anatomy. Patients with predominant annular dilatation and limited valve tethering could be the ideal candidates for annuloplasty, whereas in presence of predominant leaflet tethering, MitraClip could still represent the most appropriate therapy.

The combination of different technologies may represent an ideal option in selected FMR patients with particularly advanced tethering and LV remodeling, as has been shown in surgical experience.[17] However, if increasing clinical data continues to prove the efficacy and safety of percutaneous annuloplasty devices, it may call for a complete paradigm shift in the way FMR is treated; that is, treating FMR patients with moderate MR to prevent left atrial and ventricular dilatation, atrial fibrillation, as well as worsening MR and LV function.

REFERENCES

1. Maisano F, Alfieri O, Banai S, et al. The future of transcatheter mitral valve interventions: competitive or complementary role of repair vs. replacement? Eur Heart J 2015;36(26):1651–9.
2. Gillinov AM, Cosgrove DM, Blackstone EH, et al. Durability of mitral valve repair for degenerative disease. J Thorac Cardiovasc Surg 1998;116(5): 734–43.
3. Flameng W, Herijgers P, Bogaerts K. Recurrence of mitral valve regurgitation after mitral valve repair in degenerative valve disease. Circulation 2003; 107(12):1609–13.
4. Maisano F, La Canna G, Grimaldi A, et al. Annular-to-leaflet mismatch and the need for reductive annuloplasty in patients undergoing mitral repair for chronic mitral regurgitation due to mitral valve prolapse. Am J Cardiol 2007;99(10):1434–9.
5. Kunzelman KS, Reimink MS, Cochran RP. Annular dilatation increases stress in the mitral valve and

delays coaptation: a finite element computer model. Cardiovasc Surg 1997;5(4):427–34.

6. Votta E, Maisano F, Soncini M, et al. 3-D computational analysis of the stress distribution on the leaflets after edge-to-edge repair of mitral regurgitation. J Heart Valve Dis 2002;11(6):810–22.

7. Timek TA, Liang D, Daughters GT, et al. Effect of semi-rigid or flexible mitral ring annuloplasty on anterior leaflet three-dimensional geometry. J Heart Valve Dis 2008;17(2):149–54.

8. Jensen MO, Jensen H, Smerup M, et al. Saddle-shaped mitral valve annuloplasty rings experience lower forces compared with flat rings. Circulation 2008;118(14 Suppl):S250–5.

9. Chong CF. Are rigid annuloplasty rings better than flexible annuloplasty rings in ischemic mitral regurgitation repair: where is the evidence? Ann Thorac Surg 2009;88(6):2073 [author reply: 2073–4].

10. Bothe W, Kvitting JP, Stephens EH, et al. Effects of different annuloplasty ring types on mitral leaflet tenting area during acute myocardial ischemia. J Thorac Cardiovasc Surg 2011;141(2):345–53.

11. Maisano F, Redaelli A, Soncini M, et al. An annular prosthesis for the treatment of functional mitral regurgitation: finite element model analysis of a dog bone-shaped ring prosthesis. Ann Thorac Surg 2005;79(4):1268–75.

12. McCarthy PM, McGee EC, Rigolin VH, et al. Initial clinical experience with Myxo-ETlogix mitral valve repair ring. J Thorac Cardiovasc Surg 2008;136(1): 73–81.

13. Magne J, Pibarot P, Dumesnil JG, et al. Continued global left ventricular remodeling is not the sole mechanism responsible for the late recurrence of ischemic mitral regurgitation after restrictive annuloplasty. J Am Soc Echocardiogr 2009;22(11): 1256–64.

14. Braun J, Bax JJ, Versteegh MI, et al. Preoperative left ventricular dimensions predict reverse remodeling following restrictive mitral annuloplasty in ischemic mitral regurgitation. Eur J Cardiothorac Surg 2005;27(5):847–53.

15. Calafiore AM, Di Mauro M, Gallina S, et al. Mitral valve surgery for chronic ischemic mitral regurgitation. Ann Thorac Surg 2004;77(6):1989–97.

16. Lee AP, Acker M, Kubo SH, et al. Mechanisms of recurrent functional mitral regurgitation after mitral valve repair in nonischemic dilated cardiomyopathy: importance of distal anterior leaflet tethering. Circulation 2009;119(19):2606–14.

17. De Bonis M, Lapenna E, La Canna G, et al. Mitral valve repair for functional mitral regurgitation in end-stage dilated cardiomyopathy: role of the "edge-to-edge" technique. Circulation 2005; 112(9 Suppl):I402–8.

18. Mann DL, Kubo SH, Sabbah HN, et al. Beneficial effects of the CorCap cardiac support device:

five-year results from the Acorn Trial. J Thorac Cardiovasc Surg 2012;143(5):1036–42.

19. Bolling SF, Pagani FD, Deeb GM, et al. Intermediate-term outcome of mitral reconstruction in cardiomyopathy. J Thorac Cardiovasc Surg 1998; 115(2):381–6 [discussion: 387–8].

20. Tahta SA, Oury JH, Maxwell JM, et al. Outcome after mitral valve repair for functional ischemic mitral regurgitation. J Heart Valve Dis 2002;11(1): 11–8 [discussion: 18–9].

21. Ciarka A, Braun J, Delgado V, et al. Predictors of mitral regurgitation recurrence in patients with heart failure undergoing mitral valve annuloplasty. Am J Cardiol 2010;106(3):395–401.

22. De Bonis M, Lapenna E, Verzini A, et al. Recurrence of mitral regurgitation parallels the absence of left ventricular reverse remodeling after mitral repair in advanced dilated cardiomyopathy. Ann Thorac Surg 2008;85(3):932–9.

23. Takeda K, Sakaguchi T, Miyagawa S, et al. The extent of early left ventricular reverse remodelling is related to midterm outcomes after restrictive mitral annuloplasty in patients with non-ischaemic dilated cardiomyopathy and functional mitral regurgitation. Eur J Cardiothorac Surg 2012;41(3): 506–11.

24. Bax JJ, Braun J, Somer ST, et al. Restrictive annuloplasty and coronary revascularization in ischemic mitral regurgitation results in reverse left ventricular remodeling. Circulation 2004;110(11 Suppl 1):Ii103–8.

25. Taramasso M, Buzzatti N, La Canna G, et al. Interventional vs. surgical mitral valve therapy. Which technique for which patient? Herz 2013;38(5):460–6.

26. Maisano F, Franzen O, Baldus S, et al. Percutaneous mitral valve interventions in the real world: early and 1-year results from the ACCESS-EU, a prospective, multicenter, nonrandomized post-approval study of the MitraClip therapy in Europe. J Am Coll Cardiol 2013;62(12):1052–61.

27. Glower DD, Kar S, Trento A, et al. Percutaneous mitral valve repair for mitral regurgitation in high-risk patients: results of the EVEREST II study. J Am Coll Cardiol 2014;64(2):172–81.

28. Lim DS, Reynolds MR, Feldman T, et al. Improved functional status and quality of life in prohibitive surgical risk patients with degenerative mitral regurgitation after transcatheter mitral valve repair. J Am Coll Cardiol 2014; 64(2):182–92.

29. Taramasso M, Denti P, Buzzatti N, et al. Mitraclip therapy and surgical mitral repair in patients with moderate to severe left ventricular failure causing functional mitral regurgitation: a single-centre experience. Eur J Cardiothorac Surg 2012;42(6): 920–6.

30. De Bonis M, Lapenna E, Maisano F, et al. Long-term results (</=18 years) of the edge-to-edge

mitral valve repair without annuloplasty in degenerative mitral regurgitation: implications for the percutaneous approach. Circulation 2014;130(11 Suppl 1):S19–24.

31. Grayburn PA, Roberts BJ, Aston S, et al. Mechanism and severity of mitral regurgitation by transesophageal echocardiography in patients referred for percutaneous valve repair. Am J Cardiol 2011; 108(6):882–7.

32. Harnek J, Webb JG, Kuck KH, et al. Transcatheter implantation of the MONARC coronary sinus device for mitral regurgitation: 1-year results from the EVOLUTION phase I study (Clinical Evaluation of the Edwards Lifesciences Percutaneous Mitral Annuloplasty System for the Treatment of Mitral Regurgitation). JACC Cardiovasc Interv 2011;4(1):115–22.

33. Schofer J, Siminiak T, Haude M, et al. Percutaneous mitral annuloplasty for functional mitral regurgitation: results of the CARILLON Mitral Annuloplasty Device European Union Study. Circulation 2009; 120(4):326–33.

34. Dubreuil O, Basmadjian A, Ducharme A, et al. Percutaneous mitral valve annuloplasty for ischemic mitral regurgitation: first in man experience with a temporary implant. Catheter Cardiovasc Interv 2007;69(7):1053–61.

35. Machaalany J, St-Pierre A, Senechal M, et al. Fatal late migration of viacor percutaneous transvenous mitral annuloplasty device resulting in distal coronary venous perforation. Can J Cardiol 2013;29(1): 130.e1–4.

36. Piazza N, Bonan R. Transcatheter mitral valve repair for functional mitral regurgitation:

coronary sinus approach. J Interv Cardiol 2007; 20(6):495–508.

37. Siminiak T, Wu JC, Haude M, et al. Treatment of functional mitral regurgitation by percutaneous annuloplasty: results of the TITAN trial. Eur J Heart Fail 2012;14(8):931–8.

38. Maisano F, La Canna G, Latib A, et al. First-in-man transseptal implantation of a "surgical-like" mitral valve annuloplasty device for functional mitral regurgitation. JACC Cardiovasc Interv 2014;7(11): 1326–8.

39. Siminiak T, Dankowski R, Baszko A, et al. Percutaneous direct mitral annuloplasty using the Mitralign Bident system: description of the method and a case report. Kardiol Pol 2013; 71(12):1287–92.

40. Raman J, Jagannathan R, Chandrashekar P, et al. Can we repair the mitral valve from outside the heart? A novel extra-cardiac approach to functional mitral regurgitation. Heart Lung Circ 2011;20(3): 157–62.

41. Palacios IF, Condado JA, Brandi S, et al. Safety and feasibility of acute percutaneous septal sinus shortening: first-in-human experience. Catheter Cardiovasc Interv 2007;69(4):513–8.

42. Heuser RR, Witzel T, Dickens D, et al. Percutaneous treatment for mitral regurgitation: the QuantumCor system. J Interv Cardiol 2008;21(2): 178–82.

43. Jilaihawi H, Virmani R, Nakagawa H, et al. Mitral annular reduction with subablative therapeutic ultrasound: pre-clinical evaluation of the ReCor device. EuroIntervention 2010;6(1):54–62.

Transcatheter Mitral Valve Replacement

Ala Al-Lawati, MD, Anson Cheung, MD*

KEYWORDS

- Transcatheter mitral valve replacement • Mitral valve devices • Catheter-based therapy
- Mitral regurgitation

KEY POINTS

- Transcatheter mitral valve replacement provides a reasonable alternative in high-risk surgical patients requiring mitral valve surgery.
- Several transcatheter mitral valve devices are available. Each device has a unique design and all are undergoing extensive preclinical testing before in-human use.
- The initial experience with in-human use of this novel technique shows an acceptable rate of associated morbidity and mortality in high-risk surgical patients.
- A multidisciplinary heart team approach is recommended for assessing patients' candidacy for transcatheter mitral valve replacement.
- Patients with poor ejection fraction and inadequate ventricular reserve might not benefit from this procedure.

INTRODUCTION

Mitral valve disease prevalence is on the rise worldwide. An estimated 2% of the general population has significant mitral valve disease. Around 2 million patients in the United States are affected with moderate-to-severe mitral regurgitation (MR). Incidence increases in the elderly with a prevalence of 9% in those older than 75 years of age.[1]

Given its inherent structural complexity, mastering the whole spectrum of mitral valve surgery remains a challenge to many surgeons. In the last 2 decades, the approach to mitral valve surgery has been standardized with well-described techniques for a variety of mitral valve pathologies. Specific mitral valve repair techniques have shown great results with excellent long-term outcomes.

In recent years, several approaches to mitral valve disease have been advocated that include minimally invasive surgery and catheter-based intervention. The benefits of these approaches will remain questionable until there are long-term data showing comparable results to that of the standard open techniques. However, in the high-risk surgical group, open mitral valve surgery carries increased risk of mortality and morbidity, and in some patients the surgical risk is prohibitive. Underreferral and underutilization of mitral valve surgery and intervention has also been documented.[2] The novel intervention of transcatheter mitral valve replacement (TMVR), may provide a safer and reasonable alternative to people in this category.

The most well-studied transcatheter approach to the mitral valve is the MitraClip System (Abbott Laboratory, Abbott Park, IL, USA). The randomized, controlled endovascular valve edge-to-edge repair study (EVEREST) II trial showed comparable long-term outcomes between the 2 studied groups with regard to mortality. However, there were more residual MR cases requiring mitral valve surgery in the MitraClip

---

Dr A. Cheung is a consultant with stock option for Neovasc Inc.

Division of Cardiothoracic Surgery, St. Paul's Hospital, University of British Columbia, 1081 Burrard Street, Vancouver, British Columbia V6Z 1Y6, Canada

* Corresponding author.

E-mail address: ACheung@providencehealth.bc.ca

Intervent Cardiol Clin 5 (2016) 109–115

http://dx.doi.org/10.1016/j.iccl.2015.08.010

group at 1 and 4 years. Eligibility for MitraClip requires a very specific set of echocardiographic characteristics of the mitral valve, rendering it not suitable for many patients.[3]

TRANSCATHETER MITRAL VALVE DESIGN AND INITIAL EXPERIENCE RESULTS

Transcatheter aortic valve replacement (TAVR) underwent a significant improvement in the last few years, allowing application of some of its principles in the attempt to treat other valvular heart disease. Unlike the aortic valve, mitral valve catheter-based therapy has its unique set of challenges. For example, the mitral valve structure is far more complex than the aortic valve. There is an increased risk of damaging nearby structures with TMVR, including circumflex artery, conduction system, and aortic valve. Displacement of the anterior mitral leaflet (AML) may cause systolic anterior motion leading to left ventricular outflow tract (LVOT) obstruction. Physiologically, the mitral valve is constantly facing high systolic pressure requiring a more robust valve anchoring mechanism. Unlike aortic stenosis and TAVR, the lack of calcification of the mitral valve in MR patients indicates that radial force cannot be the sole mechanism of valve anchorage.

Himbert and colleagues,[4] and others, reported the use of the TAVR device SAPIEN XT (Edwards Lifesciences, Irvine, CA, USA) in the mitral position via a transseptal approach with promising initial results. This technique, however, relies on the presence of significant mitral annular calcification for a satisfactory anchoring of the valve in the mitral position.[4–6] The incidence of valve malpositioning, embolization, paravalvular regurgitation, and LVOT obstruction remains high.

The fundamental differences of the mitral valve require the development of a transcatheter system specific for its anatomy and disease state. These have undergone extensive studies in animal and cadaveric models. Both porcine and ovine models were used to demonstrate TMVR's feasibility and efficacy.[7–10] There are many TMVR systems with a variety of delivery methods, valve designs, and anchoring mechanisms at various stages of development and clinical trials. Some of these include CardiAQ (CardiAQ Valve Technologies, CA, USA), Tiara (Neovasc Inc, British Columbia, Canada), Edwards FORTIS (Edwards Lifesciences Corp, CA, USA), Tendyne (Tendyne Inc, MN, USA), Medtronic-TMV (Medtronic Inc, MN, USA), Highlife Medical-TMV (Highlife Medical CA, USA), Gorman-TMV (Trustee of University of

Pennsylvania, PA, USA), and Endovalve (Micro Interventional Devices, Langhome, PA, USA). These are all trileaflet self-expanding valves with nitinol-based frames. Valve anchoring is based either on axial fixation principle, outward radial force, or a combination, depending on the design. Most have features that capture the mitral leaflets and secure the valve to the mitral annulus. Many TMVR devices have additional features to address paravalvular leakage. Most manufacturers' device designs allow fine-positioning adjustment and device retrieval before the final stage of deployment, with some allowing this even after full valve deployment. Delivery approaches include transapical, transvenous-transseptal, and transatrial. Currently, transapical is the preferred access. The delivery system size ranges from 26 F to 42 F.[7–17]

The CardiAQ valve (Fig. 1) is a trileaflet bovine pericardial valve that can be delivered transapical or transvenous-transseptal. The device design has 2 sets of opposing anchors that secure the valve to the mitral annulus. The left ventricular anchors go between the native chordae to capture the native mitral leaflets and engage the mitral annulus from the ventricular side, while the left atrial anchors stabilize the prosthetic valve and prevent it from tilting or dropping below the mitral annulus.[7,11,12] In 2012, Søndergaard and colleagues[11] reported the first in-human implant of a TMVR using the first-generation CardiAQ valve. This was performed in an 86-year-old subject with severe MR with left ventricular ejection fraction (LVEF) of 40% and Society of Thoracic Surgeons' (STS) score of 31.9%. Valve deployment used a

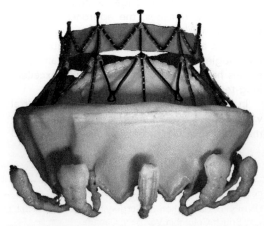

Fig. 1. Second-generation CardiAQ valve with the 2 sets of atrial and ventricular opposing anchors. (*Courtesy of* CardiAQ Valve Technologies, Irvine, CA, USA; with permission.)

ransfemoral, transseptal approach. This was done under extracorporeal circulation support as a precautionary measure because no prior experience was reported. Retrospective analysis deemed this unnecessary. The procedure was uneventful and the transcatheter valve hemodynamics were satisfactory in the immediate postoperative period. This subject died on the third postoperative day because of systemic inflammatory response and multiorgan failure. The investigators postulated the trigger being the use of an extracorporeal assist device. Postmortem examination did not reveal any device malfunction. In 2015, Søndergaard and colleagues reported their experience with the second-generation CardiAQ device using the transapical approach. All subjects had STS mortality score greater than 20%. Satisfactory device deployment and positioning was achieved in all subjects. Cardiopulmonary bypass was required in 2 subjects. There was 1 in-hospital mortality as a result of postoperative pneumonia. The 2 other subjects were discharged home and showed improved clinical and echocardiographic results on their short-term follow-up. The investigators conclude their experience by suggesting that the transapical approach may provide more flexibility and accuracy in TMV positioning and deployment compared with the transfemoral approach.[11,12] An ongoing trial to assess the valve performance as well as short-term and long-term safety outcomes of the transapical approach is being conducted in

Europe. Also, an early feasibility trial in the United States is being planned to assess both the transfemoral and transapical approach.[18,19]

The Tiara valve (Fig. 2) is a D-shaped, trileaflet bovine pericardial valve. The valve shape is designed to anatomically fit the mitral valve orifice without causing LVOT obstruction or compressing on the nearby circumflex artery. It has an atrial flange and 3 ventricular anchoring tabs that secure the valve onto the mitral annulus. Following deployment of the atrial portion, gentle traction in the direction of the left ventricle is recommended to allow adequate seating of the valve and the deployment of the ventricular tabs. During valve positioning and deployment, 2 of these anchors are aimed to capture the AML and anchor it to both trigones. Capturing the anterior leaflet by the anchor mechanism reduces the risk of postoperative systolic anterior motion of the AML. The third anchor captures the posterior leaflet and anchors it to the posterior annulus. This allows 3-point fixation of the TMV on the ventricular aspect of the native annulus and result in a very secure valve positioning. The transapical system for the Tiara valve is 32 F.[7,13,14] The authors' group in St Paul's Hospital, Vancouver, Canada, reported the first 2 in-human cases of TMVR using the Tiara valve performed early in 2014. Both subjects had severe symptomatic MR with LVEF less than 25%. Both subjects were deemed very high-risk for open mitral valve surgery by the hospital's Heart Team.

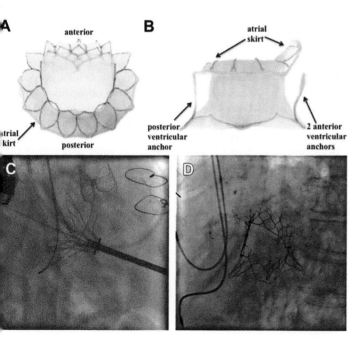

Fig. 2. Tiara valve. (A) The D-shape trileaflet valve and atrial skirt. (B) Atrial skirt and 3 ventricular anchors. (C) Deployment of the Tiara valve. (D) Postimplant Tiara valve position in a patient with an aortic valve prosthesis in situ. (Courtesy of Neovasc, Inc, Richmond, BC, Canada; with permission.)

Both procedures were done without the need for using cardiopulmonary bypass. In both cases, there was an immediate improvement in the subjects' hemodynamics with no intraoperative complications and no 30-day mortality. The valve hemodynamics at 2-month follow-up was also excellent.[13,14] A multicenter and international feasibility trial, TIARA-I is currently being conducted in Europe, United States, and Canada.[20]

The Edwards FORTIS device (Fig. 3) is a trileaflet bovine pericardial valve that is being delivered transapically through a 42 F, sheathless system. The Edwards FORTIS valve consists of a central valve body that contains the valve leaflets, an atrial flange made of nitinol struts, and 2 sets of symmetric paddles. The stent is covered on the outside with fabric to avoid injury to the native leaflets. The atrial flange is positioned at the inflow portion of the valve body and the paddles are attached to the outflow. Two of the nitinol struts in the atrial flange align to the A2 segment of the AML. These struts are designed to be more flexible, with the aim of preventing impingement on the nearby native aortic valve. The paddles' main function is to anchor the device to the native mitral leaflets and valve. The paddles can be deflected away from the valve's central body with a feature of the delivery system to capture the native mitral leaflets. Once the native mitral leaflets are captured, the delivery system is used to secure the paddles against the valve's central body, thereby anchoring the Edwards FORTIS device to the native anatomy. This allows firmer leaflet capture between the TMV and the native mitral valve. Both the atrial flange and the paddles are covered with fabric to allow future endothelialization of the prosthetic valve.[7,15] Bapat and colleagues[15] reported a case series of 5 subjects who underwent TMVR using the Edwards FORTIS device. They had satisfactory results in the immediate postprocedural assessment with minimal or no MR. Three subjects survived beyond 30 days. Their report highlights the importance of achieving complete capture of both mitral leaflets. In the presence of high closing pressures, incomplete capture of a mitral leaflet my result in device displacement and severe MR.

Another very important consideration before performing TMVR is the assessment of left ventricular reserve adequacy. The only late mortality reported in Bapat and colleagues[15] case series was a result of intractable heart failure despite satisfactory valve hemodynamics on follow-up. The authors had a very similar experience with a patient. Patients with LVEF less than 20% might not benefit from mitral valve intervention and it should be considered before contemplating TMVR in this subgroup of patients.[13]

A Tendyne valve (Fig. 4) uses the transapical approach through a 30-F delivery system. It is a self-expanding porcine pericardial valve that has a D-shaped outer valve frame that is conformable to the native mitral anatomy, with an inner frame that is circular with a large effective orifice area, and a porcine pericardial valve and unique ventricular fixation system. It has a ventricular tethering mechanism that provides constant traction of the device. The tether is affixed to an epicardial pad on the surface of the left ventricle. This system allows resheathing and repositioning capability and retrieval even after full deployment.[7,16,21] Lutter and colleagues[21] reported the first in-human use of the Tendyne valve in 2 subjects. The protocol of this trial allowed attempt of Tendyne TMV deployment in both subjects followed by a 2 hours of hemodynamic observation. A conventional mitral valve replacement was then performed after explanting the TMV. Both subjects had severe (grade 4) primary MR. Valve deployment resulted in elimination of MR in 1 subject and a residual mild (grade 1) MR in the other subject. There was no decline in the measured postprocedural cardiac output in both subjects. Following the observation period, both subjects underwent uneventful open mitral valve replacement. During the open procedure, TMV explant revealed no damage to the structure of the native mitral valve and subvalvular

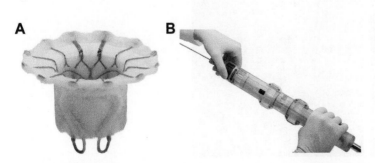

A   **B**

Fig. 3. Edwards FORTIS transcatheter mitral valve. (*A*) The valve's atrial flange, covered stent, and 2 sets of paddles. (*B*) The delivery system of Edwards FORTIS device. (*Courtesy of* Edwards Lifesciences, Irvine, CA, USA; with permission.)

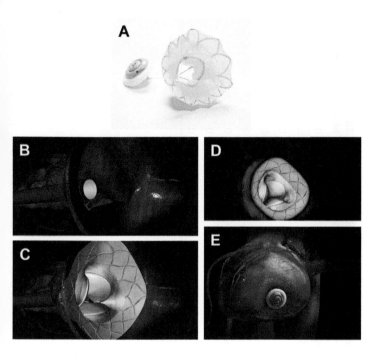

Fig. 4. Tendyne valve. (A) The self-expanding trileaflet valve with the ventricular tethering mechanism. (B & C) Deployment of the Tendyne valve. (D) Tendyne valve in mitral position after full transapical deployment. (E) The ventricular tethering mechanism that provides constant traction of the valve in mitral position after full deployment. (Courtesy of Tendyne Inc., a subsidiary of Abbott Inc.; with permission.)

apparatus. Both subjects had uncomplicated recovery. Similar to other reports, Moat and colleagues[16] reported excellent results using the Tendyne valve in 3 subjects. All 3 subjects had no intraoperative complications, were discharged home, and showed marked hemodynamic and clinical improvement on follow-up. The Tendyne mitral valve system is currently undergoing an international multicenter early feasibility trial in the United States and Australia.[22]

Medtronic transcatheter mitral valve (TMV) (Fig. 5) is designed to be delivered transatrially through the left atrium. It is a self-expanding valve that has a large atrial inflow component and a short ventricular outflow component. The atrial component allows sealing of the device and the short ventricular component minimizes the risk of LVOT obstruction. This design eliminates radial forces onto the mitral valve and valve stability is achieved instead by axial fixation. Medtronic-TMV has been extensively studied in animal models with promising results. Its in-human use is yet to be reported.[7,17]

Highlife Medical is developing a TMV that requires the use of both transatrial and transfemoral approaches. The ventricular portion has a locking component that is inserted transfemorally into the left ventricle and positioned below the native mitral annulus. The actual stent valve is delivered transatrially. It has a groove that locks to the prepositioned ventricular component. This design allows a secure anchoring and sealing of the valve into the native annulus.[7]

The previously mentioned case series show encouraging results in a very high-risk subject cohort with regard to the safety of in-human use of various TMVR devices. The 30-day mortality for all 13 subjects was 23% with some reports having zero 30-day mortality. The late mortality rate for these subjects combined was 15%. All surviving subjects showed improved functional capacity and excellent valve hemodynamics on short-term follow-up. It is worth mentioning that, despite it being high, the mortality rate is in a group of subjects with multiple comorbidities who were deemed to have either prohibitive or excessively high surgical risk. A

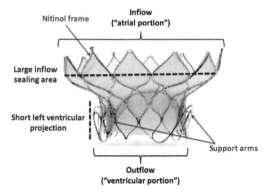

Fig. 5. Medtronic transcatheter mitral valve. (Courtesy of Medtronic, Minneapolis, MN, USA; with permission.)

Table 1
Subjects' baseline characteristics, clinical outcomes, and valve hemodynamics

	Age (y)	NYHA Class	EROA (cm²)	LVEF (%)	LVEDD (mm)	STS Score (%)	Type of Valve	Preoperative MR Grade	Type of MR	Postoperative MR Grade	Valve Gradient	NYHA Class	30-Day Mortality	Late Mortality
Cheung et al,[13] 2014	73	IV	0.59	15	76	47.7	Tiara	Severe	Functional	None	2	IV	0	1
	61	IV	0.62	25	62	4.5	Tiara	Severe	Functional	None	3	II	0	0
Søndergaard et al,[12] 2015	89	IV	0.4	55	52	36.1	CardiAQ	Severe	II	Trace	2	I	0	0
	78	IIIb	0.4	45	55	22.3	CardiAQ	Severe	IIIb	Trace	2	I	0	0
	80	IV	0.3	20	65	44.5	CardiAQ	Severe	IIIb	Trace	3	I	1	0
Moat et al,[16] 2015	68	IV	0.34	NA	NA	NA	Tendyne	Severe	Functional	None	3	Improved	0	0
	75	IV	0.79	NA	NA	NA	Tendyne	Severe	Structural	Trivial	5	Improved	0	0
	87	III	1.39	NA	NA	NA	Tendyne	Severe	Structural	None	2	Improved	0	0

Abbreviations: EROA, effective regurgitant orifice area; LLVED, left ventricular end-diastolic dimension; NA, not applicable.
Data from Refs.[12,13,16]

summary of 8 of these subjects' preoperative and postoperative characteristics are outlined in Table 1. The remaining 5 subjects, who received the Edwards FORTIS device, were not included because the valve-specific hemodynamics data are not yet published.[12,13,15,16]

SUMMARY

In summary, TMVR provides a viable and safe option in a well-selected patient population who are deemed otherwise not suitable candidates for conventional mitral valve surgery. Further experience with these devices will allow us to overcome some of the challenges associated with this technique.

REFERENCES

1. Nkomo VT, Gardin JM, Skelton TN, et al. Burden of valvular heart diseases: a population-based study. Lancet 2006;368:1005–11.
2. Mirabel M, Iung B, Baron G, et al. What are the characteristics of patients with severe, symptomatic, mitral regurgitation who are denied surgery? Eur Heart J 2003;24:1231–43.
3. Mauri L, Foster E, Glower DD, et al. 4-year results of a randomized controlled trial of percutaneous repair versus surgery for mitral regurgitation. J Am Coll Cardiol 2013;62:317–28.
4. Himbert D, Bouleti C, Iung B, et al. Transcatheter valve replacement in patients with severe mitral valve disease and annular calcification. J Am Coll Cardiol 2014;64(23):2557–8.
5. Hasan R, Mahadevan VS, Schneider H, et al. First in human transapical implantation of an inverted transcatheter aortic valve prosthesis to treat native mitral valve stenosis. Circulation 2013;128:e74–6.
6. Sinning J-M, Mellert F, Schiller W, et al. Transcatheter mitral valve replacement using a balloon-expandable prosthesis in a patient with calcified native mitral valve stenosis. Eur Heart J 2013;34:2609.
7. De Backer O, Piazza N, Banai S, et al. Percutaneous transcatheter mitral valve replacement: an overview of devices in preclinical and early clinical evaluation. Circ Cardiovasc Interv 2014;7:400–9.
8. Banai S, Jolicoeur EM, Schwartz M, et al. Tiara: a novel catheter-based mitral valve bioprosthesis: initial experiments and short-term pre-clinical results. J Am Coll Cardiol 2012;60:1430–1.
9. Lino K, Boldt J, Lozonschi L, et al. Off-pump trans-apical mitral valve replacement: evaluation after one month. Eur J Cardiothorac Surg 2012;41:512–7.
10. Banai S, Verheye S, Cheung A, et al. Transapical mitral implantation of the Tiara bioprosthesis: preclinical results. J Am Coll Cardiol Intv 2014;7:154–62.
11. Søndergaard L, De Backer O, Franzen OW, et al. First-in-Human Case of Transfemoral CardiAQ Mitral Valve Implantation. Circ Cardiovasc Interv 2015;8:e002135.
12. Søndergaard L, Brooks M, Ihlemann N, et al. Transcatheter mitral valve implantation via transapical approach: an early experience. Eur J Cardiothorac Surg 2015. pii:ezu546.
13. Cheung A, Webb J, Verheye S, et al. Short-term results of transapical mitral valve implantation for mitral regurgitation. J Am Coll Cardiol 2014;64(17):1814–9.
14. Cheung A, Stub D, Moss R, et al. Transcatheter mitral valve implantation with Tiara bioprosthesis. EuroIntervention 2014;10:U115–9.
15. Bapat V, Buellesfeld L, Peterson M, et al. Transcatheter mitral valve implantation (TMVI) using the Edwards FORTIS device. EuroIntervention 2014;10:U120–8.
16. Moat N, Duncan A, Lindsay A, et al. Transcatheter mitral valve replacement for the treatment of mitral regurgitation: in-hospital outcomes of an apically tethered device. J Am Coll Cardiol 2015;65(21):2352–3.
17. Piazza N, Bolling S, Moat N, et al. Medtronic transcatheter mitral valve replacement. EuroIntervention 2014;10:U112–4.
18. L Søndergaard. A Clinical Study of the CardiAQ™ TMVI System (Transapical DS). ClinicalTrials.gov; NLM identifier: NCT02478008.
19. Wilson Szeto, Howard Herrmann, Saibal Kar, Alfredo Trento. Early Feasibility Study of the CardiAQ™ TMVI System (Transfemoral and Transapical DS). ClinicalTrials.gov; NLM identifier: NCT02515539.
20. Raj Makkar, Martin B Leon, Stefan Verheye, Anson Cheung. Early Feasibility Study of the Neovasc Tiara Mitral Valve System (TIARA-I). ClinicalTrials.gov; NLM identifier: NCT02276547.
21. Lutter G, Lozonschi L, Ebner A, et al. First-in-human off-pump transcatheter mitral valve replacement. J Am Coll Cardiol Intv 2014;7(9):1077–8.
22. Paul Grayburn. Early Feasibility Study of the Tendyne Mitral Valve System. ClinicalTrials.gov; NLM identifier: NCT02321514.

Transcatheter Mitral Valve-in-Valve Therapy

Jose F. Condado, MD, MS, Brian Kaebnick, MD, Vasilis Babaliaros, MD*

KEYWORDS

- Valve-in-valve • Transcatheter mitral valve replacement • Mitral bioprosthesis degeneration

KEY POINTS

- Current US surgical practices favor mitral valve repair or bioprosthetic replacement over mechanical valves, especially in the growing elderly population.
- Valve-in-valve (VIV) or valve-in-ring (VIR) transcatheter mitral valve replacement (TMVR) has been used for the treatment of inoperable patients with failing mitral valve repairs or bioprosthesis.
- Procedure planning with transthoracic and transesophageal echocardiogram must be complemented with a cardiac computed tomography angiography.
- A heart team evaluation is needed for patient selection and procedure planning, including access (transapical, transseptal, transatrial) and transcatheter heart valve type and size.
- VIV-TMVR and VIR-TMVR have reported success rates of 70% to 100%.

INTRODUCTION

Transcatheter aortic valve replacement (TAVR) is now a treatment option for high-surgical risk patients with severe aortic stenosis[1–5] and for patients with failing aortic bioprosthesis[6] known as valve-in-valve (VIV)-TAVR. Though less often performed, VIV– transcatheter mitral valve replacement (TMVR) has also been described in selected inoperable patients with failing mitral bioprosthesis. This article discusses the unique technical challenges of VIV-TMVR emerging from the complex mitral valve anatomy and limitations of existing technology.

PERCUTANEOUS TREATMENT OF FAILING MITRAL BIOPROSTHESIS

Mitral valve repairs and/or bioprosthesis replacements are increasingly used instead of mechanical valves to avoid the need of life-long systemic anticoagulation, especially in elderly patients with bleeding risk factors (ie, fall risk).[7] These bioprosthetic valves can often last between 10 and 20 years, depending on the patient's age and comorbidities,[8–10] with a risk for reoperation due to valve dysfunction of 4.1%, 13.6%, 18.8%, and 23.5%, at 5, 10, 15, and 20 years, respectively.[9] Although redo surgical mitral valve replacement is possible, the mortality of surgical reintervention increases with age, comorbidities, and urgency of the procedure.[11–14] Consequently, with the increased implantation of mitral valve bioprosthesis in an aging US population with better life expectancy than ever before, the frequency of failing surgical valves in high surgical risk patients will inevitably increase. The less invasive, VIV-TMVR can be a feasible treatment option.

BIOPROSTHETIC DEGENERATION MECHANISM

For a stented bioprosthesis in the mitral position, leaflet deterioration can result from pannus formation leading to cusp tear and mitral regurgitation (MR),[15] or from leaflet calcification

Disclosures: Dr V. Babaliaros is a consultant for Edwards Lifesciences and Abbott Vascular. Dr J.F. Condado and Dr B. Kaebnick have nothing to disclose.
Division of Cardiology, Structural Heart and Valve Center, Emory University School of Medicine, Atlanta, GA, USA
* Corresponding author. Emory University Hospital F606, 1364 Clifton Road, Atlanta, GA 30322.
E-mail address: vbabali@emory.edu

leading to mitral stenosis. Acute endocarditis is another common cause of mitral bioprosthesis failure, which results from rapid destruction of leaflets and/or adjacent structures and, consequently, MR from central leak and/or paravalvular leak (PVL).

PREPROCEDURAL EVALUATION AND PLANNING

The initial diagnosis of a failing mitral bioprosthesis is made with transthoracic echocardiogram (TTE) in a patient complaining of worsening symptoms of congestive heart failure from severe mitral stenosis or regurgitation. This initial test is followed by a transesophageal echocardiogram (TEE) to characterize the cause and anatomic characteristics of the prosthesis failure (ie, differentiate between central leak or PVL).[1] Echocardiography is also used to determine left and right ventricular function, pulmonary artery systolic pressure, and presence of multivalve disease and/or infective endocarditis.

A percutaneous treatment may be chosen in patients with symptomatic bioprosthesis deterioration that are deemed inoperable after a comprehensive heart team evaluation.[1] However, before percutaneous intervention, planning is necessary to determine the access and transcatheter heart valve (THV) type and size to be used. To date, 2 commercially available THVs have been successfully used for a VIV-TMVR: the balloon-expandable SAPIEN or SAPIEN XT valve (Edwards Lifesciences, Irvine, CA, USA) and the balloon-expandable MELODY valve (Medtronic, Dublin, Ireland). The SAPIEN XT valve has bovine pericardial leaflets mounted on a cobalt chromium frame and was originally designed for implantation in the native aortic valve. The MELODY valve consists of bovine

jugular vein leaflets mounted on a platinum iridium frame and was originally designed for the pulmonary valve. The MELODY has a longer, covered stent frame that may facilitate valve deployment and prevent the occurrence of PVL; however, the SAPIEN XT valve is most commonly used because of its durability in the aortic position (including antimineralization treatment) and its larger available sizes up to 29 mm (the largest nominal MELODY size is 23.5 mm outer diameter). The Direct Flow valve (Direct Flow Medical, Santa Rosa, CA, USA) is a fully repositionable and retrievable THV with bovine pericardium leaflets that has been successfully implanted in 1 case of severe calcified mitral stenosis[16] and 1 case of mitral VIR-TMVR.[17] Unfortunately, this valve is unavailable outside clinical trials in the United States.

The THV size selection must be based on the internal diameter of the surgical valve, which must not be confused with the external diameter used to categorize the surgical bioprosthesis sizes. Oversizing the THV to the bioprosthesis can lead to underexpansion of the THV with resulting increased transvalvular gradients; and undersizing can lead to late THV embolization, significant PVL, and patient–prosthesis mismatch. Available free mobile applications (ie, Mitral VIV), based on in vitro testing of surgical and transcatheter valves diameters, can be used for valve size selection but, ultimately, a cardiac computed tomography angiography (CTA) helps to accurately calculate the real internal diameter of the bioprosthetic stent,[18] which is affected by years of pannus formation and calcification.[19] Thus, a preprocedural cardiac CTA helps determine the percutaneous access, THV size, ideal fluoroscopy angles, and risk of left ventricular outflow track obstruction after the THV deployment (**Fig. 1**).

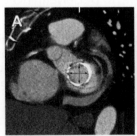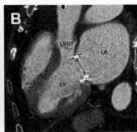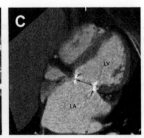

Fig. 1. Preprocedural cardiac CTA evaluation. An inoperable patient (Society of Thoracic Surgeons [STS] score 19.6%) with a failing 27 mm mitral Edwards bioprosthesis scheduled for VIV-TMVR underwent preprocedural CTA. (*A–C*) Measured internal diameters (*black arrows*) using multiple views were 25 × 25 mm. (*B*) CTA is also used to select the landing zone, by evaluating the proximity between the ventricular outflow tract (LVOT) and the mitral bioprosthesis. LVOT obstruction can happen if the transcatheter valve is deployed too far into the ventricle. Patient successfully underwent VIV-TMVR with a 26 mm SAPIEN XT valve. LA, left atrium; LV, left ventricle.

VALVE-IN-VALVE–TRANSCATHETER MITRAL VALVE REPLACEMENT

Successful cases of VIV-TMVR have been previously reported in nonsurgical candidates with failing mitral valve bioprosthesis.[20–33] VIV-TMVR can be performed using a transapical, transatrial, or transseptal approach. In a transapical approach, a small anterolateral thoracotomy in the fifth or sixth intercostal space is used to access the pericardial space and left ventricular apex, introducing the THV delivery system through it. This access type has been most commonly used because it allows direct access to the mitral apparatus and coaxial retrograde deployment of the THV within the failing surgical bioprosthesis (Fig. 2). In a transatrial approach, a small anterolateral thoracotomy is made to access the left atria for an anterograde deployment of the THV. In a transseptal approach, initial access is obtained from the femoral vein, from which the catheters and delivery system are advanced into the left atria by performing a transseptal puncture that is followed by anterograde THV deployment (Fig. 3). The transseptal approach avoids a thoracic incision, which can result in a prompt postprocedure recovery and may be preferred in patients with extremely depressed ejection fraction, severe chronic lung disease, or multiple sternotomies, in whom a transapical incision may be detrimental. In some cases, the wire can be externalized through a small apical sheath or snared in the distal aorta to provide extra stability during transseptal VIV-TMVR.

In 1 of the first case series of VIV-THV valve replacements, Webb and colleagues[21] described 7 subjects who underwent VIV-TMVR using a transseptal (n = 1), transatrial (n = 1), or transapical (n = 5) approach. Although, in this early experience, subjects implanted using a transseptal and transatrial access died due to procedural complications, later case reports and series have reported successful implantations using both approaches.[25,27,28,31,33] The initial success of the transapical VIV-TMVR has been confirmed in successive series,[23,24,28,29,34] with Cheung and colleagues describing a 5-year survival of 90.4% in a cohort of 23 subjects who underwent transapical VIV-TMVR.[23] The less invasive transseptal approach has also been successfully used in 2 cases requiring emergent transcatheter valve replacement due to failing mitral bioprosthesis.[31,33]

Once THV size selection and percutaneous access has been decided, the landing zone must be selected in the catheterization laboratory by using fluoroscopy and TEE guidance. The stented surgical bioprosthesis provides the fluoroscopic landmarks and an acceptable semirigid and circular (instead of oval) landing zone that can be used during percutaneous valve

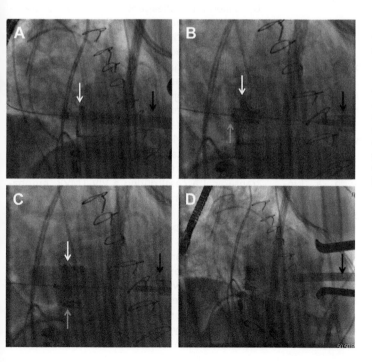

Fig. 2. Fluoroscopy of a transapical VIV-TMVR. In a patient (STS score 19.6%) with failing 27 mm Edwards bioprosthesis, (A) the delivery system was introduced using a transapical access, a 26 mm SAPIEN XT valve was (B) advanced and (C) deployed. Final fluoroscopy reveals well-positioned VIV (D). Black arrows, apical delivery system; brown arrows, SAPIEN XT valve; white arrows, surgical bioprosthesis.

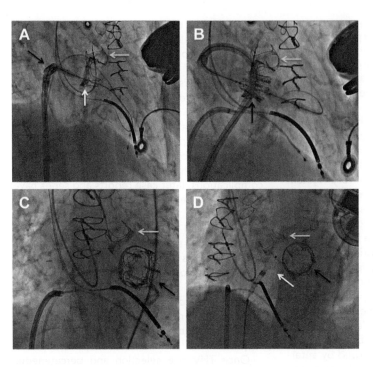

Fig. 3. Transseptal VIV-TMVR. A patient with history of aortic and mitral valve replacement (STS score 13.7%) presented with failing of the 33 mm mitral Carpentier-Edwards Perimount bioprosthesis (*white arrow*). (A) The delivery system of the transcatheter heart valve was advanced using a transseptal puncture (*black arrow*). (B) A 26-mm SAPIEN XT (Edwards Lifesciences) was deployed with the mitral bioprosthesis (*black arrow*). (C) Final fluoroscopy reveals well-positioned SAPIEN XT valve within the surgical bioprosthesis. (D) Deployment of an Amplatzer septal occluder (St. Jude Medical, Saint Paul, MN, USA) for the closure of the hemodynamically significant atrial septal defect (*green arrow*). Black arrows, SAPIEN XT valve; brown arrows, aortic bioprosthesis.

replacement. However, similar to the aortic position, this rigid landing zone can also cause underexpansion of the THV, resulting in patient prosthesis mismatch and higher than normal transvalvular pressure gradients. Typically, the THV is deployed so that the skirt is in contact with the inflow ring of the stented bioprosthesis.

VALVE-IN-RING–TRANSCATHETER MITRAL VALVE REPLACEMENT

Valve-in-ring (VIR)-TMVR is also possible in inoperable patients with recurrent mitral valve disease after repair with ring implantation.[17,26,28,35–40] VIR-TMVR is performed using the transapical, transatrial, or transseptal approaches, with the THV landing within the support of the mitral ring. Device embolization and postprocedure PVL can be an important concern because, compared with a bioprosthesis, mitral rings have a smaller landing area due to its oval morphology and shorter length. Excessive oversizing can cause annular rupture due to the absence of the semirigid stent found in surgical valves. A comprehensive heart team evaluation in an institution with experience in percutaneous treatment of structural heart disease can aid in minimizing these risks during implantation. Often, bench top testing is performed before VIR-TMVR to troubleshoot any potential complications.

COMPLICATIONS

Though VIV-TMVR or VIR-TMVR have reported successes of 70% to 100%,[21,28,30] these procedures can have severe and life-threatening complications, commonly related to the access used, and require surgical correction. In a case series by Cullen and colleagues[27] of 19 VIV transcatheter valve replacements (9 transseptal VIV-TMVRs), 4 (21.1%) subjects developed a vascular complication and 1 subject (5.2%) had a hemodynamically significant residual atrial septal defect that required device closure. In another series of 23 subjects who underwent transapical VIV-TMVR, Cheung and colleagues reported that 6 (26.1%) subjects developed major bleeding and 1 (4.3%) subject had a major stroke. Three cases of THV embolization have been reported (2 with transseptal and 1 with transapical access) during a VIV-TMVR, emphasizing the importance of landing zone and THV size selection.[21,31,32] Whereas in the aortic position THV embolization generally happens toward the aorta, in the mitral position migration can occur toward the left ventricle or the left atrium. Emergent surgery due to mitral ring dislodgement was described in 1 case of VIR-TMVR.[41] Left ventricular outflow tract obstruction is more common with VIV-TMVR and can be predicted by cardiac CTA. On-table alcohol septal ablation and TAVR with CoreValve

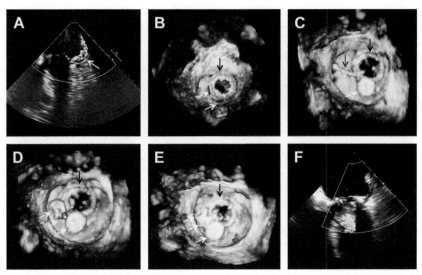

Fig. 4. PVL evaluation with TEE with Doppler and three-dimensional (3D) reconstruction. (A) Baseline Doppler revealed severe PVL (*white arrow*) with (B) 2 distinct PVL spaces on 3D reconstruction (*white arrows*). (C–E) Patient underwent transapical PVL closure using multiple 3 ventricular septal occluders and 1 vascular plug (*white arrows*). (C) Gray arrow points to catheter. (F) Final Doppler shows resolution of PVL. Black arrows point to mitral bioprosthesis.

(Medtronic) are 2 proposed solutions that have been successfully performed.

PARAVALVULAR LEAK

Mild PVL is often seen with a benign course in patients with surgical bioprosthesis.[42–44] However, in 1% to 5% of patients with PVL an intervention is needed because of regurgitation or hemolysis.[45–47] Clinically significant PVL can result from a sealing failure between the surgical bioprosthesis and the annulus (paravalvular) causing volume regurgitation, with or without concomitant central MR (ie, infective endocarditis), or as a sealing failure between the deployed THV and the surgical bioprosthesis or ring (intervalvular) after VIV-TMVR or VIR-TMVR.

Diagnosis of PVL is usually suspected after a TTE or TEE, and confirmed with a three-dimensional reconstruction TEE that further determines the location, size, and shape of the paravalvular space (Fig. 4). Echocardiographic characterization of PVL can be difficult in patients with multiple paravalvular spaces, markedly eccentric regurgitant jets, or poor echocardiographic images (either due to poor windows or presence of acoustic shadows caused by the bioprosthesis). In these cases, computed tomography can accurately determine the size and location of the PVL and may help differentiate central versus paravalvular origin. A functional cardiac MRI can estimate

the regurgitation volume and fraction, and aids in the determination of PVL severity.

Surgical treatment of clinically significant PVL consists of either valve replacement or paravalvular space closure.[48] However, transcatheter therapies are increasingly used[49–54] because open surgery has an elevated rate of PVL recurrence (12%–35%) and mortality. Percutaneous PVL closures are performed in the catheterization laboratory under general anesthesia, using a transapical, transseptal, or transaortic access.[48] The first 2 access locations have been described in the VIV-TMVR section. The transaortic access consists of advancing a catheter from the femoral artery retrograde across the aortic valve for the mitral intervention. After access is achieved, cannulation of the paravalvular space is performed under fluoroscopic and TEE guidance using a duct occluder, septal occluder, or vascular plug II (see Fig. 4). The device type is selected based on the PVL anatomic characteristics using preprocedural and intraprocedural imaging.

SUMMARY

Transcatheter mitral therapies are emerging as feasible treatment options for high surgical risk patients presenting with deterioration of prior surgical bioprosthesis or repair. A comprehensive heart team evaluation and preprocedural imaging is critical to determine the diagnosis and best therapeutic intervention. It should include a TTE, TEE, cardiac CTA, and/or functional cardiac MRI. Common transcatheter mitral therapies include VIV-TMVR, VIR-TMVR, and transcatheter PVL closure. Further studies are needed to validate these initial experiences and the role of new transcatheter devices.

REFERENCES

1. Nishimura RA, Otto CM, Bonow RO, et al. 2014 AHA/ACC guideline for the management of patients with valvular heart disease: a report of the American College of Cardiology/American Heart Association Task Force on Practice Guidelines. J Am Coll Cardiol 2014;63(22):e57–185.
2. Leon MB, Smith CR, Mack M, et al. Transcatheter aortic-valve implantation for aortic stenosis in patients who cannot undergo surgery. N Engl J Med 2010;363(17):1597–607.
3. Smith CR, Leon MB, Mack MJ, et al. Transcatheter versus surgical aortic-valve replacement in high-risk patients. N Engl J Med 2011;364(23):2187–98.
4. Popma JJ, Adams DH, Reardon MJ, et al. Transcatheter aortic valve replacement using a self-expanding bioprosthesis in patients with severe aortic stenosis at extreme risk for surgery. J Am Coll Cardiol 2014;63(19):1972–81.
5. Adams DH, Popma JJ, Reardon MJ, et al. Transcatheter aortic-valve replacement with a self-expanding prosthesis. N Engl J Med 2014;370(19):1790–8.
6. Dvir D, Webb JG, Bleiziffer S, et al. Transcatheter aortic valve implantation in failed bioprosthetic surgical valves. JAMA 2014;312(2):162–70.
7. Gammie JS, Sheng S, Griffith BP, et al. Trends in mitral valve surgery in the United States: results from the Society of Thoracic Surgeons Adult Cardiac Surgery Database. Ann Thorac Surg 2009; 87(5):1431–7 [discussion: 1437–9].
8. Chan V, Malas T, Lapierre H, et al. Reoperation of left heart valve bioprostheses according to age at implantation. Circulation 2011;124(11 Suppl):S75–80.
9. Ribeiro AH, Wender OC, de Almeida AS, et al. Comparison of clinical outcomes in patients undergoing mitral valve replacement with mechanical or biological substitutes: a 20 years cohort. BMC Cardiovasc Disord 2014;14:146.
10. Rahimtoola SH. Choice of prosthetic heart valve in adults an update. J Am Coll Cardiol 2010;55(22): 2413–26.
11. Maganti M, Rao V, Armstrong S, et al. Redo valvular surgery in elderly patients. Ann Thorac Surg 2009; 87(2):521–5.
12. Balsam LB, Grossi EA, Greenhouse DG, et al. Reoperative valve surgery in the elderly: predictors of risk and long-term survival. Ann Thorac Surg 2010; 90(4):1195–200 [discussion: 1201].
13. Jamieson WR, Burr LH, Miyagishima RT, et al. Reoperation for bioprosthetic mitral structural failure: risk assessment. Circulation 2003;108(Suppl 1):II98–102.
14. Akins CW, Buckley MJ, Daggett WM, et al. Risk of reoperative valve replacement for failed mitral and aortic bioprostheses. Ann Thorac Surg 1998; 65(6):1545–51 [discussion: 1551–2].
15. Butany J, Yu W, Silver MD, et al. Morphologic findings in explanted Hancock II porcine bioprostheses. J Heart Valve Dis 1999;8(1):4–15.
16. Mellert F, Sinning JM, Werner N, et al. First-in-man transapical mitral valve replacement using the Direct Flow Medical(R) aortic valve prosthesis. Eur Heart J 2015;36(31):2119.
17. Latib A, Montorfano M, Agricola E, et al. First-in-Human Implantation of a Direct Flow Medical Valve in a Radiolucent Mitral Annuloplasty Ring. JACC Cardiovasc Interv 2015;8(6):e105–8.
18. Jilaihawi H, Kashif M, Fontana G, et al. Cross-sectional computed tomographic assessment improves accuracy of aortic annular sizing for transcatheter aortic valve replacement and reduces the incidence of paravalvular aortic regurgitation. J Am Coll Cardiol 2012;59(14):1275–86.
19. Mylotte D, Osnabrugge RL, Martucci G, et al. Failing surgical bioprosthesis in aortic and mitral position. EuroIntervention 2013;9(Suppl):S77–83.
20. de Weger A, Tavilla G, Ng AC, et al. Successful transapical transcatheter valve implantation within a dysfunctional mitral bioprosthesis. JACC Cardiovasc Imaging 2010;3(2):222–3.
21. Webb JG, Wood DA, Ye J, et al. Transcatheter valve-in-valve implantation for failed bioprosthetic heart valves. Circulation 2010;121(16):1848–57.
22. Cheung AW, Gurvitch R, Ye J, et al. Transcatheter transapical mitral valve-in-valve implantations for a failed bioprosthesis: a case series. J Thorac Cardiovasc Surg 2011;141(3):711–5.
23. Cheung A, Webb JG, Barbanti M, et al. 5-year experience with transcatheter transapical mitral valve-in-valve implantation for bioprosthetic valve dysfunction. J Am Coll Cardiol 2013; 61(17):1759–66.
24. Seiffert M, Conradi L, Baldus S, et al. Transcatheter mitral valve-in-valve implantation in patients with degenerated bioprostheses. JACC Cardiovasc Interv 2012;5(3):341–9.
25. Montorfano M, Latib A, Chieffo A, et al. Successful percutaneous anterograde transcatheter valve-in-valve implantation in the mitral position. JACC Cardiovasc Interv 2011;4(11):1246–7.
26. Bouleti C, Fassa AA, Himbert D, et al. Transfemoral implantation of transcatheter heart valves after deterioration of mitral bioprosthesis or previous ring annuloplasty. JACC Cardiovasc Interv 2015; 8(1 Pt A):83–91.

27. Cullen MW, Cabalka AK, Alli OO, et al. Transvenous, antegrade Melody valve-in-valve implantation for bioprosthetic mitral and tricuspid valve dysfunction: a case series in children and adults. JACC Cardiovasc Interv 2013;6(6):598–605.

28. Schafer U, Bader R, Frerker C, et al. Balloon-expandable valves for degenerated mitral xenografts or failing surgical rings. EuroIntervention 2014;10(2):260–8.

29. Wilbring M, Alexiou K, Tugtekin SM, et al. Transapical transcatheter valve-in-valve implantation for deteriorated mitral valve bioprostheses. Ann Thorac Surg 2013;95(1):111–7.

30. Ferrera C, Almeria C, Maroto L, et al. Mitral valve in valve: a new choice to be still cautious. Int J Cardiol 2014;171(2):304–7.

31. Fassa AA, Himbert D, Brochet E, et al. Emergency transseptal transcatheter mitral valve-in-valve implantation. EuroIntervention 2013;9(5):636–42.

32. Cerillo AG, Chiaramonti F, Murzi M, et al. Transcatheter valve in valve implantation for failed mitral and tricuspid bioprosthesis. Catheter Cardiovasc Interv 2011;78(7):987–95.

33. Alli O, Booker O, Davies J. Emergent transcatheter mitral valve-in-valve implantation in a patient with cardiogenic shock secondary to a failed mitral bioprosthesis. Catheter Cardiovasc Interv 2015. [Epub ahead of print].

34. Cheung A, Webb J, Verheye S, et al. Short-term results of transapical transcatheter mitral valve implantation for mitral regurgitation. J Am Coll Cardiol 2014;64(17):1814–9.

35. de Weger A, Ewe SH, Delgado V, et al. First-in-man implantation of a trans-catheter aortic valve in a mitral annuloplasty ring: novel treatment modality for failed mitral valve repair. Eur J Cardiothorac Surg 2011;39(6):1054–6.

36. Petronio A, Giannini C, De Carlo M, et al. Antegrade percutaneous valve implantation for mitral ring dysfunction, a challenging case. Catheter Cardiovasc Interv 2012;80(4):700–3.

37. Mazzitelli D, Bleiziffer S, Noebauer C, et al. Transatrial antegrade approach for double mitral and tricuspid "valve-in-ring" implantation. Ann Thorac Surg 2013;95(1):e25–7.

38. Descoutures F, Himbert D, Maisano F, et al. Transcatheter valve-in-ring implantation after failure of surgical mitral repair. Eur J Cardiothorac Surg 2013;44(1):e8–15.

39. Himbert D, Brochet E, Radu C, et al. Transseptal implantation of a transcatheter heart valve in a mitral annuloplasty ring to treat mitral repair failure. Circ Cardiovasc Interv 2011;4(4):396–8.

40. Himbert D, Descoutures F, Brochet E, et al. Transvenous mitral valve replacement after failure of surgical ring annuloplasty. J Am Coll Cardiol 2012; 60(13):1205–6.

41. Descoutures F, Himbert D, Lepage L, et al. Contemporary surgical or percutaneous management of severe aortic stenosis in the elderly. Eur Heart J 2008;29(11):1410–7.

42. Ionescu A, Fraser AG, Butchart EG. Prevalence and clinical significance of incidental paraprosthetic valvar regurgitation: a prospective study using transoesophageal echocardiography. Heart 2003; 89(11):1316–21.

43. O'Rourke DJ, Palac RT, Malenka DJ, et al. Outcome of mild periprosthetic regurgitation detected by intraoperative transesophageal echocardiography. J Am Coll Cardiol 2001;38(1):163–6.

44. Genoni M, Franzen D, Vogt P, et al. Paravalvular leakage after mitral valve replacement: improved long-term survival with aggressive surgery? Eur J Cardiothorac Surg 2000;17(1):14–9.

45. Davila-Roman VG, Waggoner AD, Kennard ED, et al. Prevalence and severity of paravalvular regurgitation in the Artificial Valve Endocarditis Reduction Trial (AVERT) echocardiography study. J Am Coll Cardiol 2004;44(7):1467–72.

46. Bloch G, Vouhe PR, Menu P, et al. Long-term evaluation of bioprosthetic valves: 615 consecutive cases. Eur Heart J 1984;5(Suppl D):73–80.

47. Jindani A, Neville EM, Venn G, et al. Paraprosthetic leak: a complication of cardiac valve replacement. J Cardiovasc Surg 1991;32(4):503–8.

48. Kliger C, Eiros R, Isasti G, et al. Review of surgical prosthetic paravalvular leaks: diagnosis and catheter-based closure. Eur Heart J 2013;34(9): 638–49.

49. Sorajja P, Cabalka AK, Hagler DJ, et al. Long-term follow-up of percutaneous repair of paravalvular prosthetic regurgitation. J Am Coll Cardiol 2011; 58(21):2218–24.

50. Nietlispach F, Johnson M, Moss RR, et al. Transcatheter closure of paravalvular defects using a purpose-specific occluder. JACC Cardiovasc Interv 2010;3(7):759–65.

51. Ruiz CE, Jelnin V, Kronzon I, et al. Clinical outcomes in patients undergoing percutaneous closure of periprosthetic paravalvular leaks. J Am Coll Cardiol 2011;58(21):2210–7.

52. Cortes M, Garcia E, Garcia-Fernandez MA, et al. Usefulness of transesophageal echocardiography in percutaneous transcatheter repairs of paravalvular mitral regurgitation. Am J Cardiol 2008;101(3):382–6.

53. Pate GE, Al Zubaidi A, Chandavimol M, et al. Percutaneous closure of prosthetic paravalvular leaks: case series and review. Catheter Cardiovasc Interv 2006;68(4):528–33.

54. Garcia-Borbolla Fernandez R, Sancho Jaldon M, Calle Perez G, et al. Percutaneous treatment of mitral valve periprosthetic leakage. An alternative to high-risk surgery? Rev Esp Cardiol 2009;62(4): 438–41.

Moving?

Make sure your subscription moves with you!

To notify us of your new address, find your **Clinics Account Number** (located on your mailing label above your name), and contact customer service at:

Email: journalscustomerservice-usa@elsevier.com

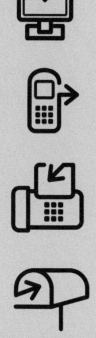

800-654-2452 (subscribers in the U.S. & Canada)
314-447-8871 (subscribers outside of the U.S. & Canada)

Fax number: 314-447-8029

Elsevier Health Sciences Division
Subscription Customer Service
3251 Riverport Lane
Maryland Heights, MO 63043

*To ensure uninterrupted delivery of your subscription, please notify us at least 4 weeks in advance of move.

Printed and bound by CPI Group (UK) Ltd, Croydon, CR0 4YY

08/05/2025

01864680-0007